Relational Gestalt Therapy in India

W0113151

This fascinating book examines the place and practice of Relational Gestalt therapy (RGT) within an Indian cultural context, and how it can be applied in a group setting.

The book begins by introducing the foundational concepts of Gestalt therapy (GT), namely phenomenology, field theory and dialogic existentialism. Through stories and vignettes, it then invites the reader to enter the circle of the group, a profound way of learning akin to the old Indian folk tradition of village communities sharing stories and bonding as a social group. Drawing from these narratives, the book not only elaborates on the theoretical concepts of GT, but also offers culturally sensitive guidance for Indian practitioners wishing to conduct group therapy.

Written by a practitioner with over 20 years' experience, this book will prove essential reading not only for practitioners working in India but also anyone with an interest in how GT can be applied in group settings in different cultural contexts.

Vanaja Ammanath has been in private practice as a therapist for the last twenty years. She has been working as a visiting faculty for Christ University, Montfort College, various government organizations, and non-government organizations in Bangalore, India, for more than two decades. As part of her ongoing education, she attended the Pacific Gestalt Institute's residential retreat in California for five years before the 2020 pandemic. As the founder of the Institute of Relational Therapy, India, she also facilitates training programs for counselors and psychotherapists in RGT. In addition to her private practice with individual clients, she has conducted group therapy for teachers, religious groups, trainee therapists, and students for over 15 years now.

The Gestalt Therapy Book Series

The Istituto di Gestalt series of Gestalt therapy books emerges from the ground of a growing interest in theory, research, and clinical practice in the Gestalt community. The members of the Scientific and Editorial Boards have been committed for many years to the process of supporting research and publications in our field: through this series we want to offer our colleagues internationally the richness of the current trends in Gestalt therapy theory and practice, underpinned by research. The goal of this series is to develop the original principles in hermeneutic terms: to articulate a relational perspective, namely a phenomenological, aesthetic, field-oriented approach to psychotherapy. It is also intended to help professions and to support a solid development and dialogue of Gestalt therapy with other psychotherapeutic methods.

The series includes original books specifically created for it, as well as translations of volumes originally published in other languages. We hope that our editorial effort will support the growth of the Gestalt therapy community; a dialogue with other modalities and disciplines; and new developments in research, clinics, and other fields where Gestalt therapy theory can be applied (e.g., organizations, education, political and social critique, and movements).

We would like to dedicate this Gestalt Therapy Book Series to all our mentors and colleagues who have sown fruitful seeds in our minds and hearts.

For a full list of titles in this series, please visit www.routledge.com/Gestalt-Therapy/book-series/GESTHE and www.gestaltitaly.com

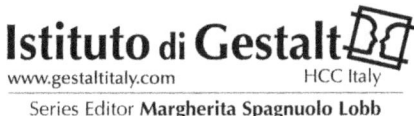

www.gestaltitaly.com   HCC Italy

Series Editor **Margherita Spagnuolo Lobb**

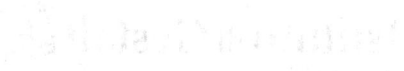

Relational Gestalt Therapy in India

A Guide to Group Practice

Vanaja Ammanath

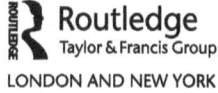

Routledge
Taylor & Francis Group

LONDON AND NEW YORK

Designed cover image: Anandi A V Nair

First published 2023
by Routledge
4 Park Square, Milton Park, Abingdon, Oxon OX14 4RN

and by Routledge
605 Third Avenue, New York, NY 10158

Routledge is an imprint of the Taylor & Francis Group, an informa business

© 2023 Vanaja Ammanath

British Library Cataloguing-in-Publication Data
A catalogue record for this book is available from the British Library

Library of Congress Cataloging-in-Publication Data
A catalog record has been requested for this book

ISBN: 978-1-032-39085-7 (hbk)
ISBN: 978-1-032-39084-0 (pbk)
ISBN: 978-1-003-34833-7 (ebk)

DOI: 10.4324/9781003348337

Typeset in Times New Roman
by Newgen Publishing UK

This book is dedicated to my mother, Valsala Ammanath, and my father, C. P. Radhakrishnan, who love me in their inimitable ways. To my teacher Friedemann Schulz, who patiently taught me Relational Gestalt Therapy over many years and continues to do so. To my students, group participants, and readers who are my guests. 'Mathru Devo Bhava, Pithru Devo Bhava, Acharya Devo Bhava, Athithi Devo Bhava' (be one for whom the Mother is God, be one for whom the Father is God, be one for whom the Teacher is God, be one for whom the Guest is God).

Contents

Acknowledgments

I will start with thanking those who paved the way for this journey of awareness and growth personally and professionally, which has led to this book.

I want to express my gratitude to Tehemtan Dhabar, Sumedha Bhise, and P. K. Saru. Each of them played a crucial role in helping me heal from my personal woundedness while generating my passion and equipping me with the skills to conduct groups experientially. Sumedha held me through some of my most challenging times and endured as my secure base for many decades.

I want to thank Marike Wusten, Charlotte Daellenbach and Elana Leigh. Each of them provided a different perspective in conducting groups. Specifically, with Charlotte, I learned to trust myself and the power of facilitating with attunement. Charlotte continues to inspire and motivate me; I am fortunate for these two decades of unswerving support, in her presence that's helped me to grow as a therapist. I also want to thank Kakli, who taught complex psychodynamic concepts with simplicity and for being a compassionate guide and supportive friend. I want to thank Nithya Purnima for meticulously going through the chapter on Indian culture, giving insightful feedback and for being my friend. I want to thank Tony Sam George for helping me understand phenomenology from a research perspective, guiding my academic growth, and being a trusting colleague.

I am grateful to Armin Bayer, Christine Campbell, Friedemann Schulz, Gary Yontef, Lynne Jacobs and Michelle Seely. They have played a significant role in helping me continue my journey with befriending my shame and supporting the development of my therapeutic skills. I want to thank Friedemann, Lynne, and Gary, for the feedback on some of the book chapters. Specifically, I want to thank Christine, for the heartwarming way she has held a space, filled with laughter and pain, for my life-changing events.

I want to thank Peter Cole, Margherita Spagnuolo Lobb and Stefania Benini for their support, feedback, and encouragement, and especially Margherita and Stefania for their consistent handholding and for sharing reading material through this process.

I want to thank my editor, Katie Randall, the copy editor and every person in Routledge—without their support and effort this book might not have seen the light of day.

I am grateful to my beloved friends Judith, Anitha, Susan, Rincy, Kathryn, Sukanto and Pinto for their support. Especially, I want to thank Kathryn, for the home away from home in Los Angeles, the warmth of her heart and hearth, margaritas, books, and fairy lights.

I also want to thank my study group with Friedemann, Jackie, Kerry and Paulina who have encouraged my writing and supported my learning with humor and warmth.

I want to thank my students, trainees, and members of all the groups I have led. I am grateful for their trust and I hope we continue to make our relational field meaningful as we satisfy and disappoint each other.

I am thankful to my sister Deepa and brother-in-law Ranjith for the books they sent, from Houston with love, to support my learning given how hard it is for me to get books on Gestalt therapy in India. My gratitude to my brother, Satish, who loves me unconditionally. Saishe, we are cut differently, but we are of the same cloth. I am grateful to my loving parents and grandparents who paved the way for my aliveness. I want to thank my partner and friend of 32 years, Venu. I think without his support it would have been challenging for me to pursue my career within my cultural context. I am grateful to our children Akamsha, Anandi and Kanna—they continue to teach me sensitivity, compassion, generosity, and on many occasions, anger management. I am grateful to my family of in-laws, they welcomed a young, scared girl from a nuclear family into their joint family and tolerated my need for space, while supporting my life in a joint family system. Especially, I want to thank Paddy, my eldest brother-in-law, who paved the way for my career in psychology through needed and valued financial support.

A special thank-you to Akamsha Ammanath for editing this book multiple times and painstaking referencing with patience and love, and to Anandi Ammanath for the cover page image.

Finally, I am grateful to my God, for this life, its opportunities, and my share of privileges.

– Vanaja Ammanath

Foreword

Margherita Spagnuolo Lobb, *Istituto di Gestalt HCC Italy*
I am honored to introduce this book, *Relational Gestalt Therapy in India: A Guide to Group Practice*. While reading it, I felt gratitude toward the author, Vanaja. As a trainer in an international school of Gestalt therapy who has worked with groups on a daily basis since 1979, I realize that this book is a significant contribution to contemporary Gestalt literature.

I find it has many merits; I will present some of them.

First, it presents Gestalt therapy work with groups in an informed way with consideration to what has been written up to this point, and contextualizes it in the contemporary world of Gestalt therapy. Despite the fact that group Gestalt therapy is the most widely known form of the Gestalt method, it is only in recent decades that significant and structured theoretical reflections on group practice have developed.

Although Fritz Perls' work with groups represented a major change in clinical method in the 1960s, his successors did not develop theoretical thinking about this innovation until the 1990s. Until then, the literature on groups was woefully sparse; books and articles on groups were few in number and did not provide a theoretical and practical structure of working in groups, which is rich in theoretical, anthropological, social, and especially clinical connotations. Looking retrospectively at this phenomenon, I have the feeling that this very innovative practice was also swallowed up in the wave of the atheoretical fashion of the 1970s–1990s, which emphasized creativity and doing at the expense of thinking and writing. Gestalt therapy *was* the in-group practice; very interesting things were happening in it, which were lost in Gestalt slogans that were not very prone to dialogue with other approaches. If for Perls the 'Californian' groups were the place of demonstration and dissemination of his new method, they also marked the birth of an original contribution to group psychotherapy in general. Group happenings were viewed in terms of figure and ground and processes, rather than content. It was Paul Goodman, however, who reflected on the group as a phenomenological and political reality and who made contributions based in a Gestalt perspective to the advancement of sociology, culture, and education (Goodman, 1942; 1956; 1972).

In the 1990s, after the deaths of Laura Perls and Isadore From, the New York Institute for Gestalt Therapy deliberately oriented its scientific interests toward groups as a viable alternative to an interest in dual dynamics (Lay & Kitzler, 1999). Their choice was based on the Gestalt concept of organism/environment field, which emphasizes that the task of psychotherapy is both private and political, in the sense that the two dimensions cannot be split (Lichtenberg, 2009). It is evident that behind a group therapy intervention there is always a thought about and passion for community, as well as an anthropological belief about social self-regulation. For a psychotherapist, working with groups is a plunge into social complexity, and it opens wide-ranging human and social horizons.

However, we had to wait until 2018 to see a book like Cole and Reese's *New Directions in Gestalt Group Therapy: Relational Ground, Authentic Self*, which, it can be said, was a watershed in the definition of the epistemological principles of Gestalt therapy with groups: an awareness of the scientific power of our work with groups and a beginning of proper Gestalt theoretical reflection that allowed us to inhabit a space of our own in the scientific literature. It is precisely to that book that Vanaja refers as the generative matrix of her reflections, offering us an informed and lively contribution to Gestalt group therapy that stems from her decades of experience with groups in India and from her academic expertise. The author has assimilated so well all that has been written in Gestalt therapy about groups that she is able to move from quoting one author to another with great fluidity, and in her words, Gestalt colleagues who have dealt with groups, including myself, are all present; all figure prominently at the right time.

But another merit of the book is the fact that Vanaja describes her application of Gestalt work with groups in a specific country, India, where the relationship between individual and society is as complex as ever. On the one hand, its colonial tradition, with its harsh imposition of rules and sanctions, creates strict control over the expression of emotions. On the other, the profoundly spiritual soul of ancient Indian culture, open to the divine within the other (the greeting namaste means just that), allows one to experience collegiality, being part of a group, as a constitutive value of existence. It is precisely India's social criticalities and the resilience given by its docile and spiritual soul, which in the silence of meditation seeks the relational meaning of things, which allows the author to apply group therapy in a restorative way with respect to the deficiencies that individual psychotherapy, with its often elitist rules, fails to resolve in that country.

The author describes how the advent of British colonization led to the loss of India's humble relationship with nature, animals, and people. Being in the world has become based on the need for power and control of the other, instead of seeking an encounter with the other as a human being in whom we can see ourselves and find meaning in our existence. Vanaja roots her work with groups in Buddhism and its philosophy of integrating man and nature. She describes the group with the symbol of the circle, in which we meet as equals and which can be found in the native cultures of many parts of the world later subjugated to power-centered cultures: the natives of North America, Australia, Mexico and the like. It was in these places that the group was used as a means to survive difficult evolutionary moments. It tells the story of Indian culture in a fluid and personal way, and it is as if we feel on our own skin the contradictions and complexities of a cultural system in which castes still prevail implicitly.

The author makes it clear that Gestalt work with groups is only possible in this type of culture if one adheres to a relational epistemology. In fact, an old-fashioned Gestalt practice centered on individual awareness, aimed at releasing unexpressed aggression, would be impossible to apply in India.

'Not many Indians are comfortable expressing their anger towards their parents, even if imaginary, and very few enjoy the idea of jumping from chair to chair giving voice to their "top dog" and "underdog"' (p. 3 (Introduction)).

Relational Gestalt therapy, on the other hand, with its phenomenology, field theory, and dialogic existentialism, can be assimilated into Indian culture. In this complex culture, the needs of people seem closer to what relational Gestalt therapy has to offer: to ally with people's intentionality in their contact, instead of breaking the habitual repression of personal wishes, thereby supporting aggression. I'd like to underline that her criticism of traditional Gestalt therapy is also criticism we can make when we consider the new clinical needs of contemporary society: it is no longer of value to support aggression as a principle per se, without considering the ground experience of our clients. We need to acknowledge that the sense of self of our clients today is more fragile and desensitized; it's in need of safe ground between them and the therapist. In this case, to express aggression might result in a destructive rather than a cathartic experience (Spagnuolo Lobb, 2020).

As Perls, Hefferline and Goodman (1994) wrote: 'The individual is at any moment inevitably part of a field, which includes both him and his environment. [...] The nature of this relationship between him and his environment determines his behavior' (p. 7 ff.). This is applied by the author to the group setting. The perspective of the group as field is distinguished from the systemic perspective: a system is observed as a separate—'other'—reality, whereas the field implies the phenomenological perspective, which answers the question 'What is my experience in this given situation?' What interests us from a field perspective is the current experience, and this can only happen at the contact boundary between the members (including the leader) and the group (Spagnuolo Lobb, 2013, p. 246). The experiences that emerge at the contact boundary in a group are not conceived as individual experiences but rather as a continuous process of being-with significant parts of the world, with excitement, determination, and choices, destructuring and reconstructing, and finally assimilating (Spagnuolo Lobb, 2018, p. 61).

Far from a dichotomous approach, the author brings to the book the language of those who know that they are interdependent with nature and other human beings, and does so with humility. In her vision of the group, the focus is not on emotions of power and control, but rather on the awareness of not being alone and the placement of the other as equal, even if different. Those who read this book will have a sense of calm and wisdom, in which the author contextualizes being in a group as both a biological and a relational function related to the survival of the species. The fact that it is written by an Indian provides added value, which fascinates the reader.

Thus, a third merit of this book is the personal, fluid, participatory, and never-detached style with which Vanaja describes the reasons she became an expert in Gestalt psychotherapy with groups in India. In keeping with what she proposes from a theoretical and clinical perspective, her narrative style is a very successful interweaving of personal accounts and clinical experiences presented within the Gestalt theoretical framework. The result for the reader is a sense of a full presence; she is there, in front of us, with all her humanity, her professionalism, and her belonging in a radical way in two communities, the Indian community and the Gestalt community.

Because of its directness, its description of the historical landscape of groups, and its look at India, this book is aimed at both early career practitioners and experts in the field. It contextualizes the work on groups in Gestalt therapy in a simple and straightforward way. It provides a cultural perspective, the Indian perspective, that allows, even for those working in the United States, as in South America or Europe or any other country, to reflect on the cultural dimension, which, if taken for granted, traps us in biases of which we are unaware. Instead, knowing different cultural realities enables us to identify more deeply and critically with our own, giving us the guidance we need to develop a cultural glance. The author herself, however, defines who should read this book: 'If bringing the self of the therapist into the relational field motivates you, if you are open to staying with uncertainties, then this book is for you' (p. 157 (Conclusion)). It is a spontaneous declaration from a phenomenological attitude. So those who are open to a humanistic, not purely technical, understanding of working with groups will find in this book an 'embodied' look, a novelty that will lead them to growth.

Vanaja loves working with groups. The passion and skill that you will perceive in her writing makes this book a useful tool for all those who work clinically with groups and who look for new knowledge of and sensitivity to relational process in group experiences. But also group leaders in general (managers, social workers, teachers, and any other practitioners of groups) can benefit from reading it and experiencing her natural *freely fluctuating leadership*, of which she is a living example.

Such a book on groups has not existed up until now, and it is a precious gift.

References

Goodman, P. (1942/1959/1977). *The Empire City*. Vintage Books.

Goodman, P. (1956/1960). *Growing up absurd*. Vintage Books.

Goodman, P. (1972). *Little prayers and finite experience*. Harper & Row.

Lay, J., & Kitzler, R. (1999). Working with group process: The model of the New York Institute for Gestalt Therapy. *Studies in Gestalt Therapy, 8*, 318–320.

Lichtenberg, P. (2009). La psicoterapia della Gestalt come rinnovamento della psicoanalisi radicale. *Quaderni di Gestalt, 12*(2), 45–68.

Perls, F., Hefferline, R., & Goodman, P. (1951/1994). *Gestalt therapy: Excitement and growth in the human personality*. Gestalt Journal Press.

Spagnuolo Lobb, M. (2013). *The now-for-next in psychotherapy. Gestalt therapy recounted in post-modern society*. Siracuse: Istituto di Gestalt HCC Italy, www.gestaltitaly.com

Spagnuolo Lobb, M. (2018). Aesthetic relational knowledge of the field: A revised concept of awareness in Gestalt therapy and contemporary psychiatry. *Gestalt Review, 22*(1): 50–68.

Spagnuolo Lobb, M. (2020). The relational turn of Gestalt therapy clinical practice: From the 'empty chair' to the 'dance of reciprocity' in the field. *International Journal of Psychotherapy, 24*(3), 17–31. https://doi.org/10.36075/IJP.2020.24.3.3/Lobb

Acronyms and Abbreviations

PHG	Perls, Hefferline and Goodman
GT	Gestalt Therapy
GGT	Gestalt Group Therapy
PGI	Pacific Gestalt Institute
ERT	Enduring Relational Themes
RGT	Relational Gestalt Therapy
NIMHANS	National Institute of Mental Health and Neuro-Science
NGOs	Nongovernmental organizations
CBT	Cognitive Behavior Therapy

Introduction

Boats at Night

For me this particular metaphor of Irvin Yalom's (1989) of boats at night captures the importance of relationality in terms of how our fear of death and isolation can become tolerable within the holding space of a caring relationship. Yalom (1989), discussing the existential anxiety about death, says that even at the point of death, the willingness of another to be fully present may penetrate the isolation. As a patient said in 'Do Not Go Gentle', 'Even though you're alone in your boat, it's always comforting to see the lights of the other boats bobbing nearby' (Yalom, 1989, p. 158).

The metaphor of lit boats has a particular meaning for me, which came up during the sharing by a member of a group therapy I conduct. I felt warm at the thought of boats around, fear of water, hope that if I drowned someone would certainly be there to rescue me, at the same time I wanted the boats to be at a comfortable distance. Too much proximity overwhelms me, pointing toward my own existential resolution of how much closeness and how much isolation I want. This particular experience of mine was evoked by the sharing of one member from a therapy group about her joy of being in groups and comparing that to lit boats. This was followed by other group members sharing the meaning they attached to the metaphor.

'I love being in groups, as a child I would go out and be mostly with neighbors and friends [...] I did not like going back home, home was a very lonely place. In groups I felt a community spirit, togetherness and warmth. When I am in a group, I can share my vulnerabilities and if in reciprocation others share their vulnerabilities, I feel connectedness and intimacy. It's like many boats in water at night, warm lights spilling out from the boats, knowing that you are not alone, there are other boats just like you [...] When that does not happen, I feel rejected [...] it brings up anger and disappointment for me'.

'The image of many boats scares me, I had numbed my senses about what a group means to me, when she spoke about the imagery of boats, I felt fear and I wanted to distance myself. For me group or community is not a safe space, I feel scared of more boats next to me, competitiveness, rivalry [...] it's threatening

DOI: 10.4324/9781003348337-1

for me, I don't know how to cope with that. I make one to one relationship even in the group. Somebody can pick on you, no one to protect you. Last four to five years I am developing a sense of—all are OK together, understanding sibling rivalry, the feeling that I am significant, I matter, and feeling protected has grown over several years'.

The experiences narrated above give an insight into how subjective experiences of the same phenomenon can vary from person to person. As a group leader, I was startled by and curious about how these unexpected revelations emerged and how it enabled a deepening of awareness for each member as well as the forging of stronger relational bonds.

As I continued to reflect on the meaning the phenomenon of group had for each member, many themes emerged. Group can be a source of comfort as well as a threat based on each individual's past experiences of groups—family, community, society. Our subjective experiences are embedded in the field, we are impacted, and we in turn impact our field. Group can foster a sense of belongingness as well as isolation. When one member expresses an experience, it can be their experience as well as that of the group members waiting for expression. When we recognize, explore with curiosity and engage in a dialogue with individual members, it expands the meaning each member holds. This develops an awareness that in turn leads to growth and change for the whole group and the larger community. Moreover, it broadens our understanding of universal existential anxieties around isolation and togetherness, and life and death.

This book is about individual experiences that get shaped in a specific cultural context. It is also about universal experiences that cut across culture and society. I bring together such individual concerns that are shaped within a cultural context which has a bearing on how we relate with ourselves and how that in turn affects therapeutic relationships. I do so specifically in the setting of group therapy, and I have tried to link these experiences to the theoretical underpinning of Relational Gestalt Therapy (RGT).

Both in paradigm and practice I am a relational Gestalt therapist. The way I facilitate a group is influenced by this. I am also informed by my psychoanalytic training in the way I understand the nuances of the dilemmas that individuals in a group struggle with. This book intends to share some of these individual dilemmas, meaning making and the importance of human connectedness while demonstrating working relationally, as much as is possible through narration. The pain of existential isolation can be addressed through connecting with oneself through an ongoing awareness process. Isolation becomes endurable and even joyful through connectedness with our environment.

I have reviewed literature relevant to RGT and combined it with the subjective experiences of my group members and myself to elucidate the application of the theory in the field of Indian culture. I believe a focus on this is vital given how our education is a legacy of our colonial past, which influences what is figural in the training of therapists. Conversations around incorporating indigenous practices into course curriculum is a phenomenon that is still in the stages of early development. Our practice is largely influenced by Western ideas of mental health, and group therapy is often conducted based on this. This book is relevant because it offers a seamless integration of Gestalt therapy (GT) with groups in India.

In India, we are facing a high demand for mental health practitioners and there is a dearth of resources that can respond to this demand. We train around 50–60 students at Master level in counseling psychology at Christ University, Bangalore, and a handful choose to continue with their education and work as therapists. Personal therapy, group therapy and supervision are part of the course requirements in some of the good institutions. However, access to experienced and trained therapists, lack of a grave understanding of how the self of the therapist impacts clients, stigma attached to seeking help, and financial constraints make it challenging for students to seek therapy. Very few trainees develop sufficient awareness, skills and competency to face the complexity of working with individual clients. Working with families, systems, groups and community, then, is a far more overwhelming experience for a novice therapist.

Group therapy provides a way to help trainees build personal and professional competency. I have also observed from my practice that often group therapy acts as a catalyst for students to overcome their trepidation to access individual therapy. Although many trainees and therapists are required to conduct groups, they find it challenging to apply the theory they have learned when they are actually faced with the ground reality of working with groups. They struggle not just with their personal sense of efficacy, but also with applying theoretical concepts to dynamic human challenges that surface in a group setting. This is further compounded by how at times the mere application of 'twin chair' and 'empty chair' learned in theory classes doesn't work. Not many Indians are comfortable expressing their anger toward their parents, even if it's imaginary, and very few enjoy the idea of jumping from chair to chair giving voice to their 'top dog' and 'underdog'. How do we then address this conundrum? There is so much more to group therapy and using gestalt techniques than what we study in college.

I intend to address some of these complex dilemmas in this book. For many years now, my students, trainees and fellow colleagues have asked me, 'how do you do it?' This book is an attempt to respond to this question. Communicate with ease, simplicity and precision how to develop 'self' of the therapist, practice inclusivity of the 'other' through attunement, be in touch with one's own enduring themes and its impact on the other and be a compassionate presence through ongoing dialogue. And when there are unavoidable disruptions and hurt in this relational bond, then we must find ways to sustain dialogue with humility and confidence. Both experiential material and theory are explicated in this book and hopefully balanced out without an overemphasis of one over the other. This book is organized in a manner that moves from the 'whole' to 'parts', at times sequentially and occasionally in a stream of consciousness. In addition, concepts from RGT are explained with examples and vignettes from work with groups.

The first Chapter, 'Circle of Belongingness', looks at the importance of groups and community and the existential need they served in human evolution in general. The circle as a metaphor and symbol of safety, intimacy and relational healing is explored and exemplified. This chapter also highlights the meaning of community, groups and society in Indian culture.

The second Chapter, 'Relational Gestalt Therapy', traces how traditional psychoanalytic practice in the West moved toward a relational stance. This is followed by history, theoretical foundations and therapeutic practice of GT and illuminates how it can be assimilated into Indian culture. Phenomenology, field theory and dialogic existentialism are explained briefly (they are further elaborated on in Chapters 6 and 7), and I have highlighted how they can be integrated with ease because of their closeness to the Indian ethos.

The third Chapter, 'Relationality and Indian Culture', looks at the complexity of giving a singular definition to Indian culture that is vastly heterogeneous while attempting to capture certain characteristics that are unique to Indian culture. I have tentatively extended certain Indian cultural characteristics through a literature review using a multidisciplinary approach. I offer an argument on how the Indian psyche is shaped and responds to a relational approach as opposed to objective neutrality or behavior modification. I have used examples from my experiences leading groups to elucidate the cultural components that resonate with a relational paradigm.

The fourth Chapter, 'Being and Becoming a Relational Therapist', presents a stance that is personal as well as gestalt, about the relevance of what the therapist brings into the relational field. The 'being' of the therapist continues to grow, change and evolve in the span of his or her professional career. This process of growth happens through the awareness the therapist is able to engage in to understand self, in terms of values, beliefs, life experiences and sociocultural context and its influences on the therapeutic bond. In that sense, and existentially speaking, the therapist's 'being' is constantly in the process of 'becoming'. There is no easy path to this process of being and becoming a compassionate, competent and skilled therapist or group leader.

The fifth Chapter, 'Framework for Facilitating Groups', offers guidelines for structuring groups with rules and norms while providing a framework that is relational. I have focused on the guidelines I use when facilitating a group, which is a combination of my theoretical orientation as well as my experiences as a group leader working in India. A vignette is provided to show how both a cultural and individual specific need for fluid time is addressed within the framework using a relational approach.

The sixth Chapter, 'Phenomenology, Field and Adjacent Possible', explains and illustrates the application of a phenomenological attitude combined with Kurt Lewin's field theory, Jan Smuts' holism and Stuart Kauffman's adjacent possible theory to the practice of group therapy. I have presented a group therapy case to illustrate the importance of not pushing one's agenda as a group leader onto members and staying in the 'here and now'. This opens up chances of adjacent possibilities and allows growth and change to happen incrementally.

Chapter 7, 'Dialogic Existentialism', discusses Martin Buber's therapeutic factors—inclusion, presence and commitment to dialogue—which is the cornerstone of RGT. Following this methodology is crucial for a therapist who wants to work relationally. Why does inclusion, presence and dialogue matter to Indians so much? This is a question which I have endeavored to answer through some case vignettes.

The eighth Chapter is on 'Enduring Relational Themes' (ERT). In this chapter, I try to explain ERTs and how they can inform our practice while working with groups. ERTs affect the way we relate to ourselves, others and our life spaces. Our themes impact and are impacted by the field. It's a personal favorite of mine and tracking it for myself and for my group members has tremendously improved the quality of my presence. It fosters the ability to engage in an ongoing exploration and dialogue to build awareness, and a case vignette from a group setting is presented to demonstrate this.

The ninth Chapter, 'Experimentation', focuses on the importance of experimentation in GT, traces its evolution and provides examples from practitioner experiences. I have also substantiated this with examples from the different groups I have conducted over the course of my work with groups. Originally there was no intention to include this chapter; however, I was deeply perturbed by the way gestalt experiments are conducted in India. Based on my limited knowledge, I have seen that often gestalt techniques like empty chair is used for behavior modification or to meet the preplanned goal of the therapist. Relational gestalt therapists give primacy to the therapeutic relationship by grounding themselves in Buber's philosophy of dialogue and on phenomenological field theory while embedding creative experiments within this relational field. I think a deeper understanding of experiments in its true intent will help practitioners be better equipped in using it judiciously and sensitively for building awareness and growth.

This book attempts to merge my instinctual ways of being present as a therapist while combining it with my learnings from my students, trainees, mentors and supervisors over the last few decades. These narratives are significant to me and my participants; they changed the way we view ourselves, others and the world. I am confident that they will be of use to you and help you reflect on your intrapsychic world, your relation to the external world, and how you engage as a group leader. I hope this book lands on you softly, seeps in gently and is soothing, easy, and simple to read—helping you be present and dialogue with yourself to make meaning of your experiences. Finally, I hope you are able to carry this self-reflection to the groups you work with.

Reference

Yalom, I. D. (1989). *Love's executioner: And other tales of psychotherapy.* Basic Books.

Chapter 1

Circle of Belongingness

Enduring Relationships

When you travel to the remote parts of India—small villages, hamlets, isolated hilly regions and forest dwellings where indigenous tribes reside—you are likely to see the enduring threads of the interrelatedness between nature and human beings. My early childhood was spent in a remote village in Kerala, in the south of India, where neither electricity nor technology had yet reached. I remember as a child being a curious observer outside the circle of women's gatherings near the village pond, men's gatherings at the local tea stall and socioreligious gatherings at the village temple during Pooram.[1] There was something fascinating about the way these group gatherings seemed to vitalize my grandparents and parents, and in turn energize me. The women would gather near the communal pond to wash clothes and bathe while narrating their daily challenges in their relationships; older women would listen and often give advice drawn from their life experiences. I would listen, fascinated as my grandmother asked questions, challenged, joked with, advised and comforted the younger women. Occasionally, I would be the enrapt outlier of my grandfather's tea-time group, where the exchanges among the men varied from world to local politics, farming tips and communal support for the needy. During Pooram, I would accompany my grandmother, mother and a small group of village women at night to watch the theater and folk-art performances. This would be organized in an open ground at the temple, and the village people would sit on straw mats spread out on the ground under the vast, star-spangled sky. Watching these dramatic performances about human struggles and the universal themes of love, anger and grief in a rustic setting created a sense of deep connection between community and nature.

Electricity reached our village during my late childhood. In the last decade or so, although technology has left its life-changing mark, some people still maintain connections to nature where trees, animals and plants are nurtured and cared for and often worshiped. A few families continue to cultivate the land in personal as well as community spaces for food requirements; the resources are shared and families support each other during periods of crisis. Annual festivities that celebrate the village deity and harvest festivals are marked by local

DOI: 10.4324/9781003348337-2

theater performances, folk music and harvest dances that are intrinsically linked to nature worship. The human need for connection still exists, even though modernization has taken away many of the group rituals.

A book on group therapy from a relational paradigm would be inadequate without a brief narrative of the interrelatedness of nature, the human existential need for connections, primal reasons for emergence of groups and the symbolic meaning of the circle from early human civilization. The existence of groups can probably be traced back to the dawn of civilization when early human beings formed small groups aimed at meeting the needs for survival, sharing, protection, belongingness and togetherness. Groups emerged as a primordial cultural phenomenon, and their healing practices were inclusive of the human relationship between individuals, with natural elements, and with the cosmos as a whole. Civilizations in general, and cultures in particular, were formed through a process of co-creation between the human being and the demands of nature into which they were born. As societies became more complex, political, religious, social and economic structures were established to organize, manage, regulate, control and protect the expanding population. These ancient cultures rightly saw their survival linked to the interrelatedness of nature, community support and the sharing of resources and knowledge.

From ancient times, 'Adivasis'[2] and other indigenous communities have gathered in circles for support, to settle disputes and for spiritual comfort. Talking circles are primitive in their origin and grounded in indigenous practices across the world. For instance, it's called *hocokah* in the Lakota language of Native Americans, meaning a sacred circle where people sit together, in prayer, to support each other's healing (Madrona, 2014). Talking circles rooted in traditional indigenous practices, by the very act of passing the 'talking feather stick', stimulated a setting for members to consciously engage in verbal expressions, receptive listening, thoughtful reflection and acceptance.

Although these rituals of talking circles were possibly practiced among the Adivasis, sadly, there is no recorded data available of this, primarily because they were inexorably pushed back into the forests and hills by the advent of other civilizations, British colonization and the post-independence era of development projects that displaced around 50 million people over the last 50 years of independence in India (Mishra, 2002; Mohanty, 2005; Singh & Ganguly, 2012; Sama, 2019; Venkitachalam et al., 2020). Loss of relationship with forests and land, loss of livelihood, poverty and the breakdown of support systems have led to appalling damage to individuals and communities in many parts of India. As civilizations continued to grow and expand, cultural traditions, language and ancient healing practices were irrevocably lost. As pointed out by ecologists and sociologists, the indigenous tribes were uprooted from their land and were driven toward extinction by the predominant cultures in power (Baldy, 2013), distancing us from healing group rituals.

Based on the published data available, the closest equivalent of a healing group in India is the 'Satsang'[3] and the 'Sangha'.[4] According to Indian academicians, the Satsang is an ancient Indian practice akin to group counseling that involves mindfulness meditation supporting spiritual and social awareness (Rybak, Sathaye, & Deuskar, 2015). The Sangha traditionally refers to the group of monks and nuns who follow the teachings of Buddha. However, the word is now also used for people who find safety and strength in a like-minded community. According to Buddhist philosophy, the pursuit of the noble eightfold path requires surrendering to the three doctrines of Buddhism, which are Buddha (enlightenment), Dharma (right action), and Sangha (community). Sangha is one of the three valued components of Buddhism, and its philosophy advocates taking refuge in the community and learning from fellow companions who support one's journey toward self-awareness and enlightenment (Khyentse & Sangye, 2006; Hanh, 1990; Rinpoche, 1998).

Man, by nature, is relational, and ongoing physical, emotional, spiritual and psychological awareness, and healing happen in relation to the other and to the larger circle of community. This indispensable yearning and survival need is a theme in the writings of Polster (2021), who is one of the most significant contributors to the field of Gestalt therapy (GT). He speaks about 'Life Focus' communities as a practice for groups that fosters in the members a sense of enchantment, belonging, vitality and continuity, which I think has always been of great import to human beings. This was a need from which we got alienated, over many decades of modernization, and today it has become critical given the pandemic situation that has left us alone in automated silos.

Communities, groups and the symbolic circle in which it gathers go back to the ancient history of human societies, cut across cultures and appear to be associated with unity, connection and personal growth through awareness. Many traditional practices and the meaning they held for ancient communities have vanished, while some symbols like the 'circle' and rituals have survived through art forms and oral folk traditions. The circle as a symbol in India is represented as a 'mandala',[5] and it is a recurring universal image (Davis, 2016). Even if the word 'mandala' may not be used as it was originally conceptualized in Sanskrit,[6] it is recognized across cultures as a collective symbol of the wholeness of the cosmos—holding connotations of integration with a higher consciousness and protection against disintegrative forces (Alpert, 1995; Dellios, 2003).

Alpert (1994) says that from a biological viewpoint, the circle is the richest in possibilities because it is evocative of the developmental calm and wholeness of the organism before polarity. As Fehr (2003) notes, the circle in which the therapy group sits is a symbolic global phenomenon that tribes and civilizations, no matter how primitive or advanced, have used in their cultures—'it's the only symbol in which all points have parity and equivalency' (p. 1). The circle in which groups usually meet can be found in cultures including communities in Native America, Africa, India, Mexico, China and Australia. In ancient times these groups served a therapeutic purpose in an informal way.

Formal History of Group Therapy

Although groups and talking circles are as ancient as human civilization and cut across all cultures, the formal psychological helping group was pioneered by Joseph Pratt in 1905, in America. Group therapy has its origins in tuberculosis sanatoria, when Pratt started a group for patients to psycho-educate them and he observed that they improved when they were encouraged to talk about their physical and emotional challenges in the group (Scheidlinger, 2004). The sheer act of talking, sharing the universality of experiences and finding a mutual understanding seemed to help patients feel better. While tracing the history of group therapy, Scheidlinger says that it continued to evolve further in the 1930s and 1940s, due especially to the psychiatric casualties of World War II who required urgent interventions.

Considerable advancements were made to the evolution of group therapy by Kurt Lewin, Fritz Perls, Carl Rogers and Irvin Yalom. By the 1960s, there was an explosion of group therapy that continued to grow with a proliferation of practices in different settings for people with schizophrenia, prison inmates, battered women, disturbed children and alcoholics. In addition, the encounter groups, primal scream and marathon groups that blossomed around this time gained quick popularity and recognition for group therapy. Eventually, the encounter groups led to alarming controversies because group leaders who lacked clinical training and the competency to ascertain warning signs, precipitated severe psychotic reactions especially in the psychologically vulnerable members (Lieberman et al., 1973). This challenged the credibility of group therapy, fueling the need to establish ethical guidelines for the practice of group therapy (Berg et al., 2017; Scheidlinger, 2004). 'Many encounter group leaders have adopted a crash program approach, successful in industry, advertising and some scientific ventures but resulting in a reductio ad absurdum in their attempts to change behaviour' (Yalom et al., 1970, p. 5).

We associate the term 'group therapy' with the exhaustive contributions of Yalom (1995) based on his extensive work with therapy groups in the last five decades. However, Perls made a seminal contribution to popularizing group therapy. Fritz and Laura Perls moved from post–World War I Germany to South Africa, then post–World War II to New York and later to California assimilating the intellectual and cultural trends of their times and disseminating their learning. They were influenced by their psychoanalytic training as well as the zeitgeist of the time, which was marked by existentialism, phenomenology and field theory. Fritz Perls was renowned for his charisma and dramatic work with individuals within a group setting, which he used to demonstrate GT to an audience. Although Perls made pioneering contributions to the development of group therapy, literature on Gestalt group therapy (GGT) is limited and his followers have tried to fill the gap through their writing (Fairfield, 2004; Feder & Ronall, 1980; Feder & Frew, 2008; Gaffney, 2010; Hodges, 2003; Kepner, 1980; Lay & Kitzler, 1999; Polster, 2021; Spagnuolo Lobb, 2012; Zinker,1980).

A comprehensive definition of group therapy includes groups used for preventing psychological illnesses, as well as for providing support, guidance, counseling and training (Barlow et al., 2004). Several professional organizations have contributed to the global discourse about group therapy, especially through the publication of journals and ethical guidelines as it has emerged from its infancy and continued to grow as a professional field (Barlow et al.; Bernard et al., 2008; Leddick, 2011).

Groups in India

The Indian joint family, where members would gather together to express themselves to an elder, the *panchayat* (local government) at the village level, Satsangs, women's groups that would gather in communal kitchens, and communal baths are all types of informal groups in India that are rooted in antiquity. These groups have been used for facilitating cohesiveness, settling grievances, promoting spiritual awareness and for cathartic expressions for minority members. According to Rybak et al. (2015), Satsang practice is similar to group counseling. The authors draw parallels between the two, saying that the process of Satsang involves three components: a leader who has attained a high level of self-awareness, individuals who are seeking the company of such a leader, and a verbal communication taking place between them. They say that Satsang in its traditional form involved listening to religious scriptures, reflecting on and integrating its meaning while encouraging compassion, mindfulness, self-awareness and self-acceptance. Frisk (2002), discussing Satsang as a growing post-Osho[7] trend in the West, describes it as a religious group where a charismatic leader gives a discourse and followers ask questions related to the problems of existence. She goes on to say that the enlightened guru occupies a special position, as they are considered as having reached ultimate spiritual realization, noting that while some gurus can respond with compassion, there are instances of mockery and possible shaming by some.

Perhaps there are commonalities between the Western concept of group therapy and the Indian concept of Satsang; however, I think equating the two may be too simplistic, from both a psychotherapeutic and a relational stance. The purpose of a Satsang is religious, with the primary intent of reading and disseminating scriptures that promote a certain way of living and connection to a higher being. Satsang by its very nature follows a guru–chela (teacher–disciple) tradition, where the hierarchies are obvious and unchallenged, the guru is seen as an evolved being, and his interpretations of the scriptures are revered explicitly. Although in principle the model of Satsang is high in its expectations for a leader, its primary focus on religion and the guru–chela attitude does not fit easily into a relational practice. Based on my reading of how group therapy was practiced by Perls, I suspect it had elements of a guru–chela relationship but as it has evolved over time, a horizontal relationship became integral to its practice. I agree with Yontef (2002) that GT is systematically relational in its underlying theory and methodology, but the relational implications in the foundational theory have not been sufficiently explained. It's only in the last few decades there has been a concerted attention toward addressing this gap.

Group therapy from a relational framework sees the group leader as a fellow companion with the group members, and the leader's experiences and expert knowledge are not seen as more valid and superior to that of the members. Yalom's (2002) conceptualization of his role as a therapist is that 'we are all in this together and there is no therapist and no person immune to the inherent tragedies of existence' (p. 8). Yalom's view of the therapist as a fellow traveler is similar to the relational gestalt therapy (RGT) premise of Martin Buber's presence and dialogue, which advocates a non-hierarchical and mutually reciprocal relationship. Yalom's and Buber's approach presumes the necessity for the group therapist to enter into a reciprocal, humble and self-disclosing relationship with the group members.

Formal group therapy in India is associated with psychiatric social workers, clinical psychologists and psychiatrists who conduct group interventions for people with substance abuse disorders, personality disorders, schizophrenia, adolescents with behavioral problems and survivors of severe trauma. Published articles related to group therapy that I could access, in an Indian setting, were related to outcome studies of brief group therapy using a cognitive behavioral approach with the above population. These usually take place in a hospital setting like the National Institute of Mental Health and Neuro-Science (NIMHANS). Over the past four decades, psychiatric social workers have been conducting group interventions, and support groups for people recovering from substance abuse and their families at NIMHANS (Ezhumalai et al., 2018). They talk about the skills required by the group therapist as well as the importance of Yalom's therapeutic factors in a group. What is lacking in these studies is a specific focus on the relational component and the cultural factors that support or hinder the group process. Researchers have argued for intervention in a group setting because there is a scarcity of resources in the country (Chatterjee et al., 2008; Singhal et al., 2018).

In Bangalore, process-oriented training groups and group therapy retreats are used in some educational settings, especially for students of counseling and nongovernmental organizations (NGOs) that offer certificate programs in counseling. In my experience as a therapist in Bangalore, I have been part of group therapy during my professional training; as a therapist I have conducted group therapy for trafficked children, students in training for counseling, teachers and religious priests and nuns.

There are no published books or articles available on group therapy with the nonclinical population, training groups or process groups in India, and there is scant research in the area of relational factors between group leaders and members. As Manickam (2010) says, this could be due to the prioritization of research in psychiatry in India, whereas research related to the psychotherapy process and relationship factors seems to have been relegated to the background.

Notes

1   Pooram: Hindu annual temple festival celebrated in Kerala often dedicated to goddesses with temple fairs, traditional folk art performances, caparisoned elephants and fireworks.
2   Adivasis: a Hindi word meaning 'original inhabitants' for the indigenous tribes of India
3   Satsang: a Sanskrit word meaning 'in the company of truth'
4   Sangha: a Pali word meaning 'community' in the Buddhist religion
5   Mandala: meaning 'container' in the Sanskrit language
6   Sanskrit: considered to be the oldest language in the world
7   Rajneesh, also known as 'Osho', was an Indian Godman, mystic and 'guru' who had avid followers across the world. He started Rajneeshpuram in Oregon, USA, and was deported in the 1980s on charges of multiple felonies.

References

Alpert, B. (1995). Cupoles, circles and mandalas. *Anthropologie, 33*(3), 171–178.
Arulmani, G. (2007). Counselling psychology in India: At the confluence of two traditions. *Applied Psychology, 56*(1), 69–82. https://doi.org/10.1111/j.1464-0597.2007.00276.x
Baldy, C. R. (2013). Why we gather: Traditional gathering in native Northwest California and the future of bio-cultural sovereignty. *Ecological Processes, 2*(1). https://doi.org/10.1186/2192-1709-2-17
Barlow, S. H., Fuhriman, A. J., & Burlingame, G. M. (2004). The history of group counseling and psychotherapy. In J. L. DeLucia-Waack, D. A. Gerrity, C. R. Kalodner, & M. T. Riva (Eds.), *Handbook of group counseling and psychotherapy* (pp. 3–22). SAGE. https://doi.org/10.4135/9781452229683.n1
Berg, R. C., Landreth, G. L., & Fall, K. A. (2017). *Group counseling: Concepts and procedures* (2nd ed.). Taylor & Francis.
Bernard, H., Burlingame, G., Flores, P., Greene, L., Joyce, A., Kobos, J. C., Leszcz, M., MacNair-Semands, R. R., Piper, W. E., McEneaney, A. M., & Feirman, D. (2008). Clinical practice guidelines for group psychotherapy. *International Journal of Group Psychotherapy, 58*(4), 455–542. https://doi.org/10.1521/ijgp.2008.58.4.455
Chatterjee, S., Chowdhary, N., Pednekar, S., Cohen, A., Andrew, G., Araya, R., Simon, G., King, M., Telles, S., Verdeli, H., Clougherty, K., Kirkwood, B., & Patel, V. (2008).

Integrating evidence-based treatments for common mental disorders in routine primary care: Feasibility and acceptability of the manas intervention in Goa, India. *World Psychiatry, 7*(1), 39–46. https://doi.org/10.1002/j.2051-5545.2008.tb00151.x

Davis, J. (2016). The primordial mandalas of East and West: Jungian and Tibetan Buddhist approaches to healing and transformation. *Neuroquantology, 14*(2). https://doi.org/10.14704/nq.2016.14.2.940

Dellios, R. (2003). (rep.). *Mandala: From sacred origins to sovereign affairs in traditional Southeast Asia* (Ser. Centre for East-West Cultural and Economic Studies, pp. 1–15). Bond University.

Fairfield, M. A. (2004). Gestalt groups revisited: A phenomenological approach. *Gestalt Review, 8*(3), 336–357. https://doi.org/10.5325/gestaltreview.8.3.0336

Feder, B., & Frew, J. (Eds.). (2008). *Beyond the hot seat revisited: Gestalt approaches to group.* Gestalt Institute of New Orleans.

Feder, B., & Ronall, R. (Eds.). (1980). *Beyond the hot seat: Gestalt approaches to group.* Brunner/Mazel.

Fehr, S. S. (2003). *Introduction to group therapy: A practical guide* (2nd ed.). Routledge.

Frisk, L. (2002). The satsang network: A growing post-Osho phenomenon. *Nova Religio, 6*(1), 64–85. https://doi.org/10.1525/nr.2002.6.1.64

Gaffney, S. (2010). *Gestalt at work: Integrating life, theory & practice.* The Gestalt Institute Press.

Hạnh, T. N. (1990). *Our appointment with life: Discourse on living happily in the present moment* (A. Laity, Trans.). Parallax Press.

Hodges, C. (2003). Creative processes in Gestalt group therapy. In M. Spagnuolo Lobb & Amendt Lyon (Eds.), *Creative license: The art of gestalt therapy* (pp. 249–259). Springer.

Kepner, E. (1980). Gestalt group process. In B. Feder & R. Ronall (Eds.), *Beyond the hot seat: Gestalt approaches to group* (pp. 5–24). Brunner/Mazel.

Khyentse, D., & Sangye, P. (2006). *The hundred verses of advice: Tibetan Buddhist teachings on what matters most.* Shambhala.

Lay, J., and Kitzler, R. (1999). Working with group process: The model of the New York Institute for Gestalt Therapy. *Studies in Gestalt Therapy, 8*, 318–320.

Leddick, G. R. (2011). The history of group counseling. In R. K. Conyne (Ed.), *The Oxford handbook of group counseling* (pp. 52–60). Oxford University Press.

Lieberman, M. A., Miles, M. B., & Yalom, I. D. (1973). *Encounter groups: First facts.* Basic Books.

Manickam, L. S. (2010). Psychotherapy in India. *Indian Journal of Psychiatry, 52*(7), 366. https://doi.org/10.4103/0019-5545.69270

Mehl-Madrona, L., & Mainguy, B. (2014). Introducing healing circles and talking circles into primary care. *The Permanente Journal, 18*(2), 4–9. https://doi.org/10.7812/tpp/13-104

Mishra, S. K. (2002). Development, displacement and rehabilitation of tribal people: A case study of Orissa. *Journal of Social Sciences, 6*(3), 197–208. https://doi.org/10.1080/09718923.2002.11892348

Mohanty, B. (2005). Displacement and rehabilitation of tribals. *Economic & Political Weekly, 40*(13), 1318–1320. https://terisas.ac.in/ckfinder/userfiles/files/ResearchPaper_SamplePaper.pdf.

Muralidhar, D., Ezhumalai, S., Dhanasekarapandian, R., & Nikketha, B. S. (2018). Group interventions. *Indian Journal of Psychiatry, 60*(8), 514. https://doi.org/10.4103/psychiatry.indianjpsychiatry_42_18

Nadimpally, S., Venkatachalam, D., & Fatima, A. (2019). *Eviction of tribals: Forced displacement and its links with poor health.* Sama: Resource Group for Women and Health. www.samawomenshealth.in/eviction-of-tribals-forced-displacement-and-its-links-with-poor-health/

Polster, E. (2021). *Enchantment and gestalt therapy: Partners in exploring life.* (M. Spagnuolo Lobb, Ed.) (Ser. Gestalt Therapy Book Series). Routledge.

Rinpoche, P. (1998). *The words of my perfect teacher: A complete translation of a classic introduction to Tibetan Buddhism.* AltaMira Press.

Rybak, C., Sathaye, D., & Deuskar, M. (2015). Group counseling and satsang: Learning from Indian group practices. *Journal for Specialists in Group Work, 40*(2), 147–162. https://doi.org/10.1080/01933922.2015.1017064

Scheidlinger, S. (2004). Group psychotherapy and related helping groups today: An overview. *American Journal of Psychotherapy, 58*(3), 265–280. https://doi.org/10.1176/appi.psychotherapy.2004.58.3.265

Singh Negi, N., & Ganguly, S. (2012, November 30). *Development projects vs. internally displaced populations in India: A literature based appraisal.* Social Science Open Access Repository. https://nbn-resolving.org/urn:nbn:de:0168-ssoar-422011

Singhal, M., Munivenkatappa, M., Kommu, J. V., & Philip, M. (2018). Efficacy of an indicated intervention program for Indian adolescents with subclinical depression. *Asian Journal of Psychiatry, 33*, 99–104. https://doi.org/10.1016/j.ajp.2018.03.007

Spagnuolo Lobb, M. (2012). La psicoterapia della Gestalt con i gruppi. Dall'esperimento di Perls in California alla scelta politica del New York Institute, fino alle moderne applicazioni [Gestalt psychotherapy with groups: From the experiment of Perls in California to the New York Institute's policy choice and modern applications]. *Quaderni di Gestalt, 25*(1), 37–49. https://doi.org/10.3280/GEST2012-001005

Venkatachalam, D., Mishra, G., Fatima, A., & Nadimpally, S. (2020). 'Marginalizing' health: Employing an equity and intersectionality frame. *Saúde em Debate, 44*, 109–119. https://doi.org/10.1590/0103-11042020s109

Yalom, I. D. (1995). *The theory and practice of group psychotherapy* (4th ed.). Basic Books.

Yalom, I. D. (2002). *The gift of therapy: An open letter to a new generation of therapists and their patients.* Harper Perennial.

Yalom, I. D., Fidle, J. W., Frank, J., Mann, J., & Sata, L. (1970). Encounter groups and psychiatry: Report of the American Psychiatric Association task force on recent developments in the use of small groups. *American Psychiatric Association, 21*(9). https://doi.org/10.1176/ps.21.9.308-b

Yontef, G. (2002). The relational attitude in Gestalt therapy theory and practice. *International Gestalt Journal, 25*(1), 15–34.

Zinker, J. C. (1980). The developmental process of a Gestalt therapy group. In B. Feder & R. Ronall (Eds.), *Beyond the hot seat: Gestalt approaches to group* (pp. 55–77). Brunner/Mazel.

Chapter 2

Relational Gestalt Therapy

My Arrival into the Circle

For a few years after my doctorate, I was a khanabadosh *(nomad)*[1]*—searching for a place I could belong to in the way I practiced as a therapist in Bangalore, India. I tried different organizations of psychology, attended conferences and sat through keynote addresses that discussed topics like transference, the application of 'Indian philosophy', yoga for mental health and cognitive behavioral therapy (CBT) as the gold standard of treatment for varying mental health issues. I felt removed from the academic circle because my way of practice was different; I rarely used CBT and classical psychoanalysis. Although I practiced yoga and followed some principles of Hindu philosophy, I seldom used it as an intervention for my clients, unless they showed an avid interest in it. I preferred focusing on the relationship with my clients and our subjective experiences of our sociocultural context, rather than specific tools and techniques. I saw the therapeutic relationship as a 'microcosm' of the world as experienced by both my client and me.*

By chance and determined research, I found out about the Pacific Gestalt Institute (PGI, California) residential retreat. I corresponded with Lynne Jacobs (cofounder, PGI) and after exchanging a few tentative emails, our correspondence resulted in my first residential retreat. Ironically, it was here I found my circle of belongingness. Although the differences in color, race and our ways of thinking were apparent with my peers and faculty, the differences stayed mostly in the ground for me. What stood out as figural was my sense of connection in the relational field that the PGI community had created. I was curious to understand the 'other', as they were to understand me. I found the community to be interested, welcoming and respectful of differences. I approached my experience with an attitude of explorative wonder, trepidation and nascent excitement. I slowly assimilated my experience over the following days, iterating my felt sense of belongingness. This developing affinity proved to be the catalyst that drew me toward RGT.

I remember my personal work during the group process with Gary Yontef (cofounder of PGI), where I shared with him my feelings of hurt with the

DOI: 10.4324/9781003348337-3

feedback he gave me during live supervision. I had volunteered to play the role of therapist in the breakout group with great nervousness, as I was the only Indian in an all-white group. At that moment I was acutely aware of my otherness—my nationality, professional training, color, gender and the complexity of my cultural identity. I was unsure whether my client would be comfortable with me and I wasn't particularly comfortable with my client. Post the session, Gary gave me feedback about what I could have done differently and I reframed that in my head, hearing only that I didn't do anything well. I decided to share this experience with some trepidation the next day in the group process, and Armin Bayer (co-facilitator) warmly supported the risk I was taking.

I don't recollect all that transpired in my personal work with Gary; however, I remember his willingness to understand my experience, his acknowledgment of my feelings in a non-defensive manner, and his sharing of remorse at the hurt I felt. I think, in that moment, we co-created a relational experience where the different layers of my isolation and shame started loosening their hold over me. The closest I can describe that experience is by quoting Rumi,[2] 'Out beyond ideas of wrongdoing and rightdoing there is a field. I will meet you there'. We managed to meet at a place that seemed beyond hierarchy, age, gender and racial difference, specifically in that order, because my social conditioning made giving feedback to a teacher and elder unthinkable.

As the retreat progressed, I was pleasantly surprised and relieved that there were no 'empty chairs' or any other techniques that I associated with GT. I have nothing against chairs, of course. There have even been times in my personal therapy where I found the use of the empty chair and twin chair techniques helpful. I have used it with my clients in the early years of my practice, although my style of work has changed since. The experimentations by the faculty and peers during the process work emerged in the moment spontaneously. The focus was on human connections, sensitivity and inclusion in the relationship between therapist and group members, and among the members as well. There was a resonance with my own natural style of practice where the focus was on the therapeutic relationship as it developed over the course of therapy and the healing power of emotional attunement.

This attentiveness to the therapeutic relationship has emerged in the practice of psychotherapy over many decades. In the humanistic existential school, the therapeutic relationship and relationality have been important since its inception. Laura Perls (1992) argued that all suffering is born within a relationship, and I think relational therapists across different schools of thought today would agree that healing is also possible within a relationship. Spagnuolo Lobb (2017), while stressing the criticality of the therapeutic relationship and the therapist's attunement to the client, uses the phrase 'aesthetic relational knowing' to describe how we learn about our client through our felt senses. I think this aesthetic relational knowing is what caregivers communicate to the infant. As parents we feel through our senses what our child is trying to express. Accumulated moments of misattunement contribute to trauma, and the therapist's ability to feel for the client supports healing.

Movement toward Relational Psychotherapy

Psychoanalysis is considered the First Force in the field of therapy and psychotherapy; it is recognized today as having its genesis in Freud's inspiring and fundamental contribution. However, long before his pivotal contributions gained fame, his followers moved away from their allegiance to classical thought, giving their own formulations of personality development, mental health and the practice of psychotherapy. Traditional psychotherapy was used with individual clients and focused on treating the client's intrapsychic conflicts without due consideration of the environmental context. Over time, therapists saw the limitations in this method. A significant reason for this was that Freud's biological deterministic approach with its focus on intrapsychic conflicts did not give primacy to the impact relationships had on the development of human personality. Especially the critical impact of the environment on personality development—early relational experiences, family, sociopolitical context and culture. In the 1950s, with the influences brought on by phenomenology, field theory and existentialism, there was a movement in psychotherapy toward overcoming these dichotomies. This allowed an integration of body and mental experiences along with the individual's relationship with society (Spagnuolo Lobb, 2016a).

During the 1950s, the psychoanalytic school started moving away from the classical Freudian approach of drive theory and toward early relationships with significant others and its impact on personality development. Seminal contributions were made by object relations theorists like Melanie Klein, Donald Winnicott and Ronald Fairbairn; ego psychologists like Edith Jacobson and Margaret Mahler; interpersonal theorists like Harry Stack Sullivan; and self-psychology theorists like Heinz Kohut and Erik Erikson (Mitchell & Black, 1995; Summers,1994; Stolorow, Brandchaft, & Atwood, 1987). These branches of the psychoanalytic school provided the impetus to look at how early experiences with significant caregivers shape the client's relationships in adult life. These post-Freudian schools harnessed the findings from studies on infant development (Spitz, 1945; Bretherton, 1992), to argue that from birth infants are interacting with the 'other'. They postulated that the infant's sense of self, ego formation and emotional self-regulation get shaped in the reciprocal interactions between the caregiver and the infant. Recent research in the field of neurobiology supports this conceptualization that early relational experiences regulate the biobehavioral system through complex neurochemical activity in the brain, which helps develop an implicit relational knowing (Stern, 2010, as cited in Ammaniti & Ferrari, 2013).

The psychoanalysts engaged in understanding the impact of relational experiences on child development, although varied in their conceptualizations, extended the common argument that the robust development of the self requires emotional attunement and responsiveness from the significant caregiver. This environment builds the capacity of the infant to regulate their emotions, wants and needs in relation to the other, thus developing the capacity to be in relationships. It supports self needs while sustaining relational bonds as the infant continues to grow into adulthood. Based on these findings, the therapeutic relationship became a significant area of focus to understand the client's presenting struggles. Considerable attention was directed to the relationship between client and therapist that played a role in the therapeutic bond, ruptures, repair and emotionally corrective experience (Alexander, 1946). Classical psychoanalysis became dynamic, where the focus expanded to include not just an analysis of the client's intrapsychic conflicts but also the dynamic interplay of individual and environment.

However, psychoanalysts continued to maintain the client as the central figure—the one whose personality and resulting distress needed to be understood, transference worked with and insight facilitated. A shift into earnestly reflecting on what the therapist brings into the field occurred over the last three decades, with the development of the intersubjective branch of the psychodynamic school that arose in America (Stolorow, Brandchaft, & Atwood; Stolorow, 2002; Stolorow, 2008). They incorporated concepts from phenomenology, field theory and existentialism that helped propel psychoanalytic thinking from a singular intrapsychic quarrying to a dyadic relational field. Intersubjective theory is a post-Cartesian dialogical psychodynamic perspective, which postulates that experience is mutually shaped between the therapist and client in the therapeutic relationship, and that psychological phenomena can be understood only in the irreducible relational context in which they take shape (Orange, Atwood, & Stolorow, 1997; Stolorow & Atwood, 1996; Stolorow, 2013). The intersubjective and relational psychoanalytic theorists moved away from an objective, neutral analyst stance to a subjective, relational stance that held the client's experiences as equally valid as that of the therapist. Mitchell (1984) talks about this as a shift in psychoanalytic theory, 'from a framework in which drives and their derivatives are understood to constitute the basic stuff of mental life, to one in which the primary ingredients are relational configurations, past and present, real and imaginary' (p. 473).

Interestingly, this focus on the relationship in psychotherapy, and the movement away from analytic neutrality and objectivity developed around seven decades ago with the advent of the humanistic-existential school. During the 1940s and 1950s, the Second and Third Force of psychotherapy, the cognitive behavioral and the humanistic-existential schools, emerged as a challenge to psychoanalysis. GT, which falls under the humanistic-existential school, was founded by Fritz Perls, Laura Perls and Paul Goodman. GT was deeply influenced by the zeitgeist of the time—the culture, art, science, politics and psychology (Gaffney, 2010; Yontef, 1993; Yontef & Fuhr, 2005; Yontef

& Jacobs, 2005; Wulf, 1996). It started as a revision of psychoanalysis and established itself formally as an integrative practice on the foundation of phenomenology, field theory and dialogic existentialism with the publication of *PHG* (1951). *PHG* was written by the founders of GT chiefly to dissolve the neurotic dichotomies (Spagnuolo Lobb & Caccamo, 2013) prevailing at that time, and it developed in the specific sociocultural context that influenced the practice of psychotherapy. I resonate with their stance that for us to understand, postulate and support the development of our knowledge and practice, we need to ground it meaningfully in our historical roots. I think it is important for us to make sense of the practice that prevailed and developed at that time in tandem with sociocultural changes, while looking at our practice today and how it needs to adapt to the changing needs of our society.

I want to stress another important movement in the practice of psychotherapy that took place during the 1950s which supported this movement— the family system perspective, which looked at the family environment in which the client's problems developed. Some of the critical factors that contributed to this shift included, research and advancement in the fields of family therapy, social work, the child guidance movement, the impact of the two World Wars on the human psyche, and Lewin's field theory (Nichols & Schwartz, 2001). These perspectives and movements relocated the responsibility for the problems and the focus of treatment from the internal world of the individual client to the entire system of family, society and cultural groups. The prior models advocated a linear causality for understanding human distress, whereas the systems model looked at a circular causality that emphasized the reciprocal and dynamic nature of relationships.

This shift and expansion in psychotherapy discourse and the resulting synergy of different schools of thought has offered exciting opportunities for us to work relationally toward better therapeutic outcomes. In the last few decades, some schools of psychotherapy in the West have emphasized relationality and highlighted how the experiences of the therapist and client can play a role in forming and sustaining a relational bond (Hargaden & Sills, 2001; Jacobs, 1991, 2004; Mitchell, 1984; Mitchell & Black, 1995; Spagnuolo Lobb, 2017; Stolorow & Atwood, 1996; Yontef, 2002; Yontef & Schulz, 2016).

This inexorable movement toward a relational approach in the practice of psychotherapy has left a mark on the practice of both individual and group therapy. Therapists from various schools of psychotherapy have practiced group therapy along with individual therapy because of the benefits the two provide when used conjointly. However, the focus on the relationship between the leader and group members has depended on the theoretical orientation from which group therapy is practiced by individual practitioners. In this context, it is important to understand the history and theoretical underpinning of GT and its embeddedness in relationality. I believe this will inform group therapists to look at how the application of GT with groups has changed over time, and I think it will help us improve our practice, especially in its applicational value to the Indian cultural context.

Gestalt Therapy

In both traditional psychoanalytic therapy and CBT, the therapist was seen as the expert physician who, either through neutral presence and interpretations, or directive challenges and disputations, acted as a change agent to help clients develop a better quality of life. This Newtonian and Cartesian approach to the patient's problems did not leave much scope for understanding the various forces in the field, both past and present, that interact with each other and co-create both impact and outcome in therapy. I believe that the already existing hierarchy of a therapist–client relationship was reinforced with this approach, and the patient's awareness, subjective experiences and sense of agency were discounted. The advent of the humanistic school and GT brought a fresh perspective by validating the phenomenological experiences of both the client and therapist, thus countering the hierarchy.

The publication of *PHG* acted as a catalyst toward valuing embodied experience and horizontal relationship—the focus shifted from the therapist's expertise to the client's phenomenology and agency. The client was seen as having the capacity to explore their awareness, and they had the creative capacity to find solutions to their problems. According to Yontef (2002), the Gestalt therapist shunned neutrality and practiced personal involvement to support awareness, creativity, spontaneity, freedom and responsibility of the client. The theoretical foundations of GT postulated by PHG provided the subsequent practitioners the impetus to focus on relationality. I will briefly describe the theoretical foundations below and will elaborate these in chapters 6 and 7.

Theoretical Foundation

Yontef, one of the foremost contributors to RGT, has asserted that a complete system of psychotherapy requires three elements: a theory of consciousness, a scientific theory and a theory of the therapeutic relationship (Schulz, 2013). According to Yontef, in GT the theory of consciousness is phenomenology; the scientific theory is the field theory, and the theory of therapeutic relationship is Buber's dialogic existentialism.

Phenomenology. Phenomenology is the study of phenomena as they appear to the subject who is experiencing them, and this is the focus of interest to the Gestalt therapist (Brownell, 2016). This approach looks at understanding the experience of the person who is experiencing the phenomena. It operates from the assumption that each being makes meaning of their experiences in their unique, subjective way. The therapist is attentive to the immediate experience where emphasis is on the emotional, sensory and bodily processes of self and client. In RGT, the phenomenological experiences of the client and therapist are seen as equally valid, thus rejecting the Cartesian subject–object divide (Jacobs, 2001; Yontef, 1993, 2002). When we apply this concept to the practice of GGT, then the experiences of each group member and the leader are equally valid. The group leader is attentive to their own phenomenology as it emerges in the moment, while being attuned to and supportive of the self-regulation of each member as it shapes the experiences of the whole group. The group is a phenomenological field in which each member's experiences are shaped, the Gestalt of the experiences of the members is co-created through a process of self-regulation, and the leader must not impose a particular course, but must simply favor the spontaneity of the processes (Spagnuolo Lobb & Caccamo, 2013). The group leader needs to observe, describe and explore the group members' experiences and bracket the need to interpret.

To be able to do this requires a fair level of competency to park our pre-formed theoretical ideas and be mindful of what emerges in the group moment to moment. I agree with Cole and Reese (2017) that mindfully staying with the embodied experiences of self and group members yields a richer result than relying purely on preformed theoretical explanations. To give an example, in 2019, I had been conducting a therapy group for more than a year where a reasonable amount of cohesiveness and trust had been established in the group's development. However, when the coronavirus pandemic hit us, it impacted all of us in different ways. The government declared an overnight lockdown, which disrupted work and living conditions, and our group therapy meetings were shifted to an online format. For many sessions, we were in touch with the instability, uncertainty, fear and shock this caused in different degrees for us. Our world had changed suddenly from face-to-face meetings to online, leading to a sudden interruption. Bloom (2020) and Spagnuolo Lobb (2020) talk about how the coronavirus was a disruption of the contact boundary that is the fulcrum from which our experiences emerge. 'The contact-boundary between therapist and patient is the place of the therapy. Treatment for us does not consist in analysis, but in the relational recognition of that intentionality of contact that had been blocked' (Spagnuolo Lobb, 2020, p. 342). The group members and I felt this block in contact as our predictable and meaningful ways of relating with each other suddenly became impossible.

The relationship that was established in our therapy group was shaken and the members were expressive of their fears. One member in particular was consistent in the sharing of their ambivalence about online sessions. Although they turned up for all the sessions, they shared their dilemma about wanting to be part of the group, and their frustrations surrounding the loss of direct human contact. We felt the loss of face-to-face sessions, while also feeling grateful that the group continued as a space for exploring the feelings that the pandemic brought up. I believe that the shift to an online medium challenged the normative stages of group development and dynamics, disrupted our contact and relationality, and brought a period of chaos in the group that had initially formed a cohesiveness.

What helped us continue despite this period of crisis was to stay with the experiences the pandemic brought up for us to which each of us had our unique responses and to cope with the uncertainty by finding new ways of establishing contact. While affirming each member's experiences, staying with the despair rather than moving into hope prematurely, we also developed rituals of virtual contact. Although, as a leader I had knowledge about the stages of group development and dynamics, the pandemic really helped me gain a deeper understanding into staying with varying subjectivities. As a group we were able to acknowledge the loss of normalcy and move, at times lithely and at times quite limply, with the uncertainty and chaos.

Field Theory. The physicist Michael Faraday coined the term 'field' to refer to the magnetic action wherein a region in the vicinity of a magnet was affected by some unobservable force. Field theory was developed further by James Maxwell, and consolidated by Albert Einstein's theory of relativity, which significantly changed the Newtonian scientific worldview by stating that there are mutually influencing forces that act upon each other (Schulz, 2013). Friedemann Schulz goes on to explain how this concept of field theory from science was applied to psychology by Gestalt psychologists Max Wertheimer, Wolfgang Köhler, Kurt Koffka and social psychologist Lewin to explain how human beings and the environment interact with and influence each other. Perls was influenced by field theory. Although he did not elaborate on it with the depth that Lewin did, he conceived the human being as an organism–environment entity, not just an organism in an environment (Perls, 1969; Brownell, 2016). 'To look at an organism itself amounts to looking upon it as an artificially isolated unit, whereas there is always an inter-dependency of the organism and its environment' (Perls, 1969, p. 38). According to Staemmler (2006), PHG, when referring to the organism/environment field, was discouraging an isolationist view of human behavior. Staemmler says that the attempt to apply field theory to understanding human behavior has led to a Babylonian confusion because it is difficult to comprehend the notion of the word 'field' in psychology, as it requires an understanding of a new paradigm.

Although it is not easy to grasp as a concept, I appreciate the effort that's been put in by Gestalt writers like Malcolm Parlett, Frank Staemmler, Schulz, Yontef, Jacobs and Margherita Spagnuolo Lobb to explain the concept of Gestalt therapy field theory. O'Neill (2008) says that it has not been well understood, discussed or applied to practice even though it is a core philosophical underpinning of GT. I agree with Parlett and Lee (2005) that the word 'field' can cause potential challenges since it can include anything and everything, loaded with different meanings and used interchangeably. I will try to focus on explaining field theory based on how Lewin transferred this scientific concept to the understanding of complex human experiences.

The fundamental postulate of Lewin's field theory was that human behavior should be understood as a function of the interaction between an individual and their experience of the environment (Parlett, 1991; Schulz, 2013; Spagnuolo Lobb, 2016b, 2018). Applied to GGT, this refers to the phenomenological field co-created between the therapist and client, as well as the field conditions that shaped their personality. This is inclusive of early childhood experiences, the sociocultural context into which each was born and developed, and the effect of this in the 'here and now' life spaces of the members. All events in the field emerge from the interaction between all the participants and their unique ways of experiencing and responding to their field conditions (Schulz, 2013; Yontef, 1993). I agree with Spagnuolo Lobb (2018) that from a Gestalt viewpoint, the question 'What do you feel?' cannot be understood at an exclusively individual level, instead it should be seen and made meaning of as a field experience, which includes the feelings of all the members.

I believe that Lewin's theory provides a robust framework for GGT, because it values the interrelatedness of the members of the group, how each impacts the other, and the larger social system that the group is part of. I appreciate the way Hodges (2003) explains this when he says that a group is a Gestalt, in terms of it having figure and ground, wholes and parts, processes and events, forces and constraints, Gestalt formation and destruction. Based on my work with groups, I resonate with him that everything that becomes figural in the group emerges from the ground of the group and that whatever comes as a figure for a group member in their emotions, emerges out of the ground of the group. For example, when one group member expresses their disappointment with me, they can often be giving voice to the group's/other members' experiences that are not getting verbalized. It is necessary then for me, as a leader, to explore this further primarily because each individual member develops awareness in relation to the other members, and the group itself grows and evolves in relation to the members (Cole & Reese, 2017). This systematic web of relationships is mutually influential, and when the individual reaches their full potential, the group as a living entity grows and it enriches the society that the members are a part of. The group leader supports this process through dialogue.

Dialogic Existentialism. Buber's dialogic existentialism is the fundamental pillar that supports and informs the therapeutic relationship in GT, whether we work with individuals or groups. Buber was a Hasidic scholar and his ideas on dialogue are built on the Jewish tradition of engagement in dialogue with another human being, which was akin to engaging in a dialogue with God (Jacobs, 1991, 1998). Buber (Buber, 1991; Buber & Agassi, 1999) talked about healing through meeting while referring to a particular kind of subject-to-subject meeting that he called the I-Thou meeting. He distinguished between two modes of meeting, which he termed the I-Thou and I-It. Schulz (2004) says that often these concepts are seen as fixed relational positions, but the

I-Thou and I-It are better seen as being extreme points on a relational spectrum. The I-Thou refers to a way of seeing and meeting the other as a subject. The I-It refers to a way of relating to the other person as an object.

From his philosophy, RGT has assimilated the three principles of inclusion, presence and commitment to dialogue (Fairfield, 2010; Hycner, 1993; Hycner & Jacobs, 1995; Jacobs, 1991; Yontef, 1993). Inclusion is akin to empathy, where the therapist steps into the experience of the client to get an embodied sense of what the client may be experiencing. This also requires the ability to step out and reflect back to the client this felt sense. Presence involves the therapist's ability to be vulnerable, authentic and real in the therapeutic encounter. Commitment to dialogue in therapy means that as therapists we engage in the therapeutic task by contacting the client as the client is, using our sensory functions for a meaningful exchange. An ongoing dialogue helps us create a space within which the client's emergent awareness, acceptance of self and sense of agency can be explored. A dialogic attitude involves care and curiosity for an exploration of how we impact each other, whether positively or negatively.

GGT is a practice where dialogic existentialism can be used effectively between the leader and group members. This requires us to have an inclusive stance toward different members of the group—respecting cultural differences like race, age, gender, religion, region, caste and sexual orientation. This includes a willingness to engage in contact and dialogue with each member in their personal context, while also cocreating a field for respecting diversity (Cole & Reese, 2017). I agree with Spagnuolo Lobb and Caccamo (2013) that our therapeutic work with groups requires us to tailor our approach through inclusion and presence that is based on the unique developmental needs of the individuals in the group, the developmental needs of the group as a whole, and the ability to be curious to the novelty and diversity of each group member. This is particularly relevant in the diverse cultural context that we work with in India, given our heterogeneous cultural characteristics.

Traditional GT, especially as practiced by Perls, has been accused of being confrontative and causing 'iatrogenic' harm to the client (Yontef & Simkin, 1989). However, RGT has made a concerted effort to develop a theory and practice that is mindful of the damage a hierarchical expert stance can cause. Awareness of what is happening for each person engaged in the dialogue, developing a moment-to-moment mindfulness, and reflecting on this is an important aspect of GGT. For us to appreciate how GGT has evolved according to the requirements of our dynamic society, we need to look at the major currents that regulated the course of its evolution.

Gestalt Group Therapy

Perls' work with individuals within a group setting was innovative given the dyadic form of psychotherapy that existed at that time. Spagnuolo Lobb and

Caccamo (2013) say that he was openly critical of individual therapy, and that his pioneering ideas in the practice of psychotherapy addressed a dissident analyst's fatigue with the dual analytic model. Elaine Kepner (1980) says that the original goal of Gestalt workshops in the 1950s was to train therapists in the theory and methods of GT as it's applied to individual therapy. She goes on to explain this further that Fritz and Laura Perls invented this form of experiential learning, believing that a method which stressed the phenomenology of the 'here and now' needed to be experienced in the here and now. At that time, the participants in these workshops were either practicing therapists or advanced graduate students from the mental health field. Many had knowledge of theories of psychotherapy, but competency and experience in working with a client in a real-life situation were limited. GGT as practiced by Fritz Perls provided a 'felt experience' of how to practice as a Gestalt therapist. While working with individuals in a group setting, he discovered how individual stories of members influenced each other and created a therapeutic effect on the whole group. Perls postulated that the individual is an inevitable part of his field and his behavior is determined by the nature of the relationship between him and his environment (PHG, 1951, p. 7). He acknowledged the contribution of Lewin's theory to GT; however, his style and focus of working with groups was individual focused.

Kepner explains the rationale for the way Perls worked in groups, and I agree with her that his model of one-to-one therapy in a group setting had a justification beyond that of his personal preference. As Laura Perls (1992) says, his intention was to demonstrate GT to professionals of psychotherapy—it was one of the infinite possibilities of using GT. She adds that, unfortunately, the techniques got associated with GT, causing confusion and harm in the way it got incorporated into all kinds of group practice like bodywork and GT, sensitivity training and GT, transactional analysis and GT, and so on, without an understanding of GT's underlying philosophy. Yalom (1995), commenting on Perls' leadership style, observes that, unwittingly, his approach became a paradox because in philosophy he advocated individual responsibility; however, his dramatic style did not often facilitate this. Unknowingly, he paved the way for a process where the substance often got mistaken for the essence of GT. Yalom, in critiquing Perls, also talks about how he was a profound thinker and contributed vastly to human existential concerns that was holistic: 'his work rests on the basic assumption of such great thinkers as Husserl, Heidegger and Sartre' (1995, p. 444). He says that contemporary GT has moved toward a more balanced approach and uses experiments in a judicious manner.

I agree that traditional GGT had its limitations in terms of overlooking the phenomenology of the client as well as the group members, and that as Yontef (1993) says, it had its pitfalls because the group leader and group would often persuade a member to emote without developing an awareness of the struggle between wanting to express and not express. Paradoxically, this pushed the client to change before sufficient awareness was developed. The way group therapy was practiced by traditional Gestalt therapists starting with Perls was quite different from the way it has evolved over the last six decades, and how it is practiced now.

Spagnuolo Lobb and Caccamo (2013) say that it was in the 1980s and 1990s that Perls' groundbreaking ideas were developed further theoretically by his followers. While tracing the history of GGT, they talk about the contribution of the Gestalt Institute of Cleveland, the New York Institute of Gestalt Therapy and the European trends that advanced Perls' innovative ideas. Until the 1980s, the most important contribution to GGT was by the Cleveland Institute, particularly Kepner, who was a pioneer of the humanistic perspective. Kepner (1980), Joseph Zinker (1991), Erving and Miriam Polster (1999), and Ed Nevis (2014) made significant contributions to the development of GGT. Kepner describes the Gestalt group process, which integrates the principles and practice of GT, as introduced by PHG and Lewin's field theory. Lewin's experience and observations led to his conceptualization that a group is more than the sum of its parts. He observed that the relational style of group members with each other led to positive changes in stuck Gestalts, especially if old behaviors were destabilized through group interactions.

Spagnuolo Lobb and Caccamo say that from the 1990s on, after the death of Laura Perls, the New York Institute of Gestalt Therapy, where GT was founded, has deliberately directed its gaze toward groups as a valid alternative to focusing singularly on dyadic dynamics (Lay & Kitzler, 1999, as cited in Spagnuolo Lobb & Caccamo, 2013). Some of the primary contributors to this are Richard Kitzler, Bud Feder, Margherita Spagnuolo Lobb and Carl Hodges. Their contribution to the development of Perls' and Lewin's ideas in the context of Gestalt group process is extensive. They developed the theoretical concepts of organism/environment connection, the importance of presence, figure/ground, whole/parts, forces/constraints, fluid leadership, and an aesthetic perspective to look at here-and-now phenomena of the group members, to name a few. Substantial contributions have been made by Hodges to GGT through the application of the concepts of Gestalt psychology field theory like figure and ground, whole and parts, strengths and constraints, and formation and destruction. I agree with Hodges (2003) that when we work in groups, 'we become aware of a global whole of which we are all a part' (p. 250).

While exploring these different currents that have enriched GGT, Spagnuolo Lobb and Caccamo (2013) talk about how these trends are also observed in European studies where there is a growing interest in peer Gestalt group models, because our formation takes place fundamentally in social groups, and also because of changes in the sociocultural context. They say that in the 1950s, the group was a container and a driving force for the individuation of the single members, who found in it the permission to have those experiences of self-fulfillment that were hindered by social norms. They talk about the sociocultural shifts where there's a movement from the individualistic to the relational and vertical perspective to the horizontal group dimension. While looking at contributions made specifically to the culture-sensitive application of GT to groups, I found noteworthy contributions by Gaffney (2010) and Bar-Yoseph (2005), who have developed a deeper understanding of cultural sensitivity while working with diverse groups in organizational settings.

We can see that GGT has become increasingly geared toward creating a learning environment to develop individual, interpersonal, social and cultural awareness. At a personal level, the individual is supported to gain awareness into what shaped their subjective experiences, and how this influences them now. At an interpersonal level, the group becomes a setting to understand relational dynamics, and at a social and cultural level, the group creates an impetus for starting a dialogue to understand and accept differences, thus providing an opportunity for communal intimacy. Contemporary GGT has assimilated classical GT principles and combined it with a relational approach for the ongoing development of a sensitive and dynamic approach to working with groups as it adapts to the changing sociopolitical landscape.

The group has increasingly become an important modality to support both individual healing and social change. In a study conducted to look at the practice patterns of Gestalt therapists in leading groups, including therapy, training, supervision, organizational development and educational groups, 101 therapists were surveyed (Feder & Frew, 2006). The review revealed that the group continues to be a popular and important modality among Gestalt therapists, particularly in conducting therapy, training and supervision activities. The shift away from a purely hot seat approach, popular in the 1950s, has continued and group leaders are relying on a blend of approaches that draw on interpersonal and systems-level interventions. The survey respondents also indicated that group support was the most important curative factor in current Gestalt therapy groups.

While reflecting on these findings, and the ideas extended by GGT practitioners, I found it thought provoking in general and specifically in the context of the changes taking place in India, and the diaspora of Indians in Europe and America. The importance of groups and a community-oriented way of relating has seeped into Indian culture, yet the sense of loss and loneliness is a theme for the present generation Indians living in mechanistic, globalized culture. For Indians in general, loss of connections and of a relationship to community and nature has become a pervasive experience. Based on my work with individuals and groups, my sense is that Indian society, which had a collectivistic bend, is moving toward an individualistic perspective, bringing with it strengths as well as challenges. The relational trends in the GGT approach may be able to address this in ways that facilitate a development of strengths, while finding creative ways to sustain social connections that are getting disrupted.

Proximity of RGT to the Indian Ethos

GT, being assimilative, was greatly influenced by Eastern philosophy, especially Zen Buddhism and mindfulness practice (Cole & Reese, 2017; Yontef & Jacobs, 2005; Wulf, 1996). GT concepts like organismic self-regulation, focusing on awareness process, paradoxical theory of change, thrownness and agency have a deep-rooted philosophy that combines existential and Buddhist philosophy. The GT concept of organismic self-regulation and awareness is defined as the individual's ability to be in touch with thoughts, feelings and actions, and the ability to regulate them. *Samma-sati* (Gard, 1963) is a mindfulness meditation that focuses on the awareness of our different senses, bodily experiences, thought processes, feelings and dharma (right action). In addition, there is great emphasis in *Samma-sati* to become aware of the awareness process itself, without allowing shame, dejection or attempts to change or interrupt the process. In the practice of right mindfulness, the mind is trained to remain in the present—open, quiet and alert. All judgments and interpretations as, when, and if they occur, must be merely registered and then suspended (Bodhi, 1994). We can see a resonance of this in GT's paradoxical theory of change. The paradox is that the more one attempts to change oneself from a position of self-rejection, the more one remains stuck. Awareness and acceptance of self and all the parts of self, including the rejected parts, is the goal of GT, and change is seen as a by-product of this process. These concepts are close to some of the philosophical streams of thought from Buddhism and Hinduism that have influenced Indian culture.

GT's focus on the experience of the client, field theory and primacy to the therapeutic relationship can be easily assimilated to Indian culture, which is marked by diversity and relationality. Within an Indian cultural context, aside from neutrality or objective disputations of irrational thinking, even the traditional GT approaches of twin chair, empty chair or dramatic enactments rarely work unless they're embedded in a strong relational alliance between the therapist and client. The client may comply; however, this compliance may often stem from wanting to conform because the therapist is an authority figure. In this context, a dialogic attitude is fundamental to the practice because it helps the leader and group members engage in a process of exploration of the hierarchies in the relational field.

Indians, in general, like to explore the meaning of life and death and have a quest to search for the meaning of their existence. They understand the concept of responsibility, thrownness and agency in the context of dharma and karma. Karma in Hindu and Buddhist philosophy refers to our fate that is a given, what we are born with and into. Dharma is the code—our agency in engaging in the right action, which can have an impact on our karma.

This is similar to Heidegger's existential concept of 'thrownness and agency' (Wheeler, 2011). Thrownness is what we are born into and have no choice in, like one's birth into a particular family, caste, religion and sociocultural environment. Agency is the existential belief that all of us have a choice about how we live this life and as adults we are responsible for the choices we make. An example would be the Indian caste system that was, and continues to be an intangible yet rigid structure one is born into. However, we have the agency to question the inequities of this system, recognize how it influences the way we treat people, and engage in the right action that involves respect and equity.

GT is useful in reflecting on the here-and-now experiences of the leader and members in the therapeutic field and the way these experiences have been shaped by the sociocultural and political context. In my work with groups, I have found that the explorations of members' experiences in the field contribute richly to the development of the therapeutic relationship as well as awareness. With many of my participants who have experienced the ill effects of hierarchy and their cultural memberships, the here-and-now question of 'how do you feel about this, as you share this with me?'—'me' being a member of a different and privileged cultural membership—has in itself led to a shift in the group dynamics while opening a window into our own feelings as a therapist.

I remember raising the question around belongingness with an Indian Muslim male who was one of the few male members in a group of Indian Hindu women and men that I facilitated. His initial response was that he was comfortable; however, he came back to the next group meeting and shared his need to belong and not offend the group or me, or have us treat him differently because of his religion. As I continued to explore this experience with him, he recollected forgotten memories from his childhood about exclusion, being teased and bullied at school and in neighborhoods where the majority were Hindus. As a therapist, I remember experiencing shame and pain when he narrated his story, shame about my privileged cultural identity as an upper-middle-class Hindu woman. Pain at the image of a vulnerable little boy being bullied. A sharing of our respective embodied experiences of anguish created a moment of deep connection for us and the group members. They were able to share their experiences of privileges and discriminations respective to their cultural memberships. These human interactions, willingness to dialogue and the use of reflective self-disclosure can be a connecting 'corrective emotional experience' (Hartman & Zimberoff, 2004) for the group.

When we make figural what we sense in the ground, we open up the opportunities to work with shaming experiences that are often shaped in the sociocultural systems that we are part of. Furthermore, this gives an opportunity for us to explore our privileges, power imbalances, internalized biases and prejudices—our own shame as therapists surrounding these prejudices and its influence on our work.

Notes

1 *Khanabadosh* is an Indian word with Farsi origins. It literally means people who carry their home on their shoulder. Nomads.
2 Jalal Ad-Din Muhammad Rumi was a thirteenth-century Persian theologian, poet and Sufi mystic.

References

Alexander, F., & French, T. M. (1946). The principle of corrective emotional experience. In *Psychoanalytic therapy: Principles and application* (pp. 66–70). Ronald Press.

Ammaniti, M., & Ferrari, P. (2013). Vitality affects in Daniel Stern's thinking: A psychological and neurobiological perspective. *Infant Mental Health Journal, 34*(5), 367–375. https://doi.org/10.1002/imhj.21405

Bar-Yoseph, T. L. (Ed.). (2005). *The bridge: Dialogues across cultures.* Gestalt Institute Press.

Bloom, D. (2020). Intentionality: The fabric of relationality. *The Humanistic Psychologist, 48*(4), 389–396. https://doi.org/10.1037/hum0000212

Bodhi, B. (Ed.). (1994). *The discourse on right view: The Sammaditthi Sutta and its commentary.* (B. Ñanamoli, Trans.). The Buddhist Publication Society.

Bretherton, I. (1992). The origins of attachment theory: John Bowlby and Mary Ainsworth. *Developmental Psychology, 28*(5), 759–775. https://doi.org/10.1037/0012-1649.28.5.759

Brownell, P. (2016). Contemporary Gestalt therapy. In D. J. Cain, K. Keenan, & S. Rubin (Eds.), *Humanistic psychotherapies: Handbook of research and practice* (pp. 219–250). American Psychological Association.

Buber, M. (1991). *Tales of the Hasidim.* Schocken Books.

Buber, M., Agassi, B. J., & Roazen, P. (1999). *Martin Buber on psychology and psychotherapy: Essays, letters, and dialogue.* Syracuse University Press.

Cole, P. H., & Reese, D. A. (2017). *New directions in gestalt group therapy: Relational ground, authentic self* (1st ed.). Routledge.

Fairfield, M. (2010). Dialogue in complex systems: The hermeneutical attitude. In L. Jacobs & R. Hycner (Eds.), *Relational approaches in gestalt therapy* (pp. 190–193). Routledge.

Feder, B., & Frew, J. E. (2006). A survey of the practice of gestalt group therapy: A second encore presentation. *Gestalt Review, 10*(3), 242–248. https://doi.org/10.5325/gestaltreview.10.3.0242

Frew, J. E. (1997). A gestalt therapy theory application to the practice of group leadership. *Gestalt Review, 1*(2), 131–149. https://doi.org/10.2307/44394034

Gaffney, S. (2010). Gestalt at work: Integrating life, theory and practice. In A. Maclean (Ed.), *Gestalt at work: Integrating life, theory & practice – Volume I.* Gestalt Institute Press.

Gard, R. A. (Ed.). (1963). *Buddhism: Great religions of modern man.* Washington Square Press.

Hargaden, H., & Sills, C. (2001). Deconfusion of the child ego state: A relational perspective. *Transactional Analysis Journal, 31*(1), 55–70. https://doi.org/10.1177/036215370103100107

Hartman, D., & Zimberoff, D. (2004). Corrective emotional experience in the therapeutic process. *Journal of Heart-Centred Therapy, 7*(2), 3–84.

Hodges, C. (2003). Creative processes in gestalt group therapy. In M. S. Spagnuolo Lobb & N. Amendt-Lyon (Eds.), *Creative License*, (pp. 249–259). Springer.

Hycner, R. H. (1993). *Between person and person: Toward a dialogical psychotherapy.* Gestalt Journal Press.

Jacobs, L. (1991, October). *The therapist as 'other:' The patient's search for relatedness* [Conference presentation]. Martin Buber's contribution to the humanities. https://secureservercdn.net/50.62.174.80/y1a.e81.myftpupload.com/wp-content/uploads/2021/09/therapist_asothers.pdf.

Jacobs, L. (1998, March). *Dialogue and Paradox* [Lecture-discussion transcript]. Captured at the Portland Gestalt Therapy Training Institute. https://secureservercdn.net/50.62.174.80/y1a.e81.myftpupload.com/wp-content/uploads/2021/09/dialogue_and_paradox.pdf

Jacobs, L. (2001). Pathways to a relational worldview. In M. R. Goldfried (Ed.), *How therapists change: Personal and professional reflections* (pp. 271–287). American Psychological Association. https://doi.org/10.1037/10392-015

Jacobs, L. (2004). Ethics of context and field: The practices of care, inclusion and openness to dialogue. In R. G. Lee (Ed.), *The values of connection: A relational approach to ethics* (pp. 35–56). Gestalt Press.

Jacobs, L. R., & Hycner, R. (1995). The dialogic ground. In *The healing relationship in gestalt therapy: A dialogic-self psychology approach* (pp. 3–29). Gestalt Journal Press.

Kepner, E. (1980). Gestalt group process. In B. Feder & R. Ronall (Eds.), *Beyond the hot seat: Gestalt approaches to group* (pp. 5–24). Brunner/Mazel.

Lay, J., & Kitzler, R. (1999). Working with group process: The model of the New York Institute for Gestalt Therapy. *Studies in Gestalt Therapy, 8*, 318–320.

Levine, B. (1979). *Group psychotherapy: Practice and development.* Prentice-Hall.

Mitchell, S. A. (1984). Object relations theories and the developmental tilt. *Contemporary Psychoanalysis, 20*(4), 473–499. https://doi.org/10.1080/00107530.1984.10745749

Mitchell, S. A., & Black, M. (1995). *Freud and beyond: A history of modern psychoanalytic thought.* Basic Books.

Nevis, E. C. (Ed.). (2014). *Gestalt therapy: Perspectives and applications.* CRC Press.

Nichols, M. P., & Schwartz, R. C. (2001). *Family therapy: Concepts and methods.* Allyn and Bacon.

O'Neill, B. (2008). Relativistic quantum field theory: Implications for gestalt therapy. *Gestalt Review, 12*(1), 7–23. https://doi.org/10.5325/gestaltreview.12.1.0007

Orange, D. M., Atwood, G. E., & Stolorow, R. D. (1997). Intersubjectivity theory and the clinical exchange. In *Working intersubjectively: Contextualism in psychoanalytic practice* (pp. 3–18). Analytic Press.

Parlett, M. (1991). Reflections on field theory. *The British Gestalt Journal, 1*, 68–91. www.elementsuk.com/libraryofarticles/fieldtheory.pdf.

Parlett, M., & Lee, R. G. (2005). Contemporary gestalt therapy: Field theory. In A. L. Woldt & S. M. Toman (Eds.), *Gestalt therapy: History, theory, and practice* (pp. 41–63). SAGE.

Perls, F. S. (1969). *Ego, hunger and aggression: The beginning of gestalt therapy.* Random House.

Perls, F. S., Hefferline, R. F., & Goodman, P. (1951). *Gestalt therapy: Excitement and growth in the human personality*. Dell.

Perls, L. (1992). *Living at the boundary*. (J. Wysong, Ed.). Gestalt Journal Press.

Polster, E., & Polster, M. (1999). *From the radical center: The heart of gestalt therapy*. Gestalt Press.

Schulz, F. (2004). *Relational Gestalt Therapy: Theoretical foundations and dialogical elements*. Pacific Gestalt Institute. https://secureservercdn.net/50.62.174.80/y1a.e81. myftpupload.com/wp-content/uploads/2021/09/RelationalGestaltTherapy.pdf.

Schulz, F. (2013). Roots and shoots of gestalt therapy field theory: Historical and theoretical developments. *Gestalt Journal of Australia and New Zealand, 10*(1), 24–47.

Schulz, F., & Yontef, G. (2016). Dialogue and experiment. *British Gestalt Journal, 25*(1), 9–21.

Spagnuolo Lobb, M. (2016a). Psychotherapy in post modern society. *Gestalt Today Malta, 1*(1), 97–113. www.gestaltitaly.com/wp-content/uploads/2017/03/Lobb-Evolution-of-Soc-and-Psychoth-May-5-16.pdf.

Spagnuolo Lobb, M. (2016b). Self as contact, contact as self: A contribution to ground experience in gestalt therapy theory of self. In J.-M. Robine (Ed.), *Self: A poliphony of contemporary gestalt therapists* (pp. 261–289). L'Exprimerie.

Spagnuolo Lobb, M. (2017). From losses of ego functions to the dance steps between psychotherapist and client: Phenomenology and aesthetics of contact in the psychotherapeutic field. *British Gestalt Journal, 26*(1), 28–37. www.academia.edu/33670 012/From_losses_of_ego_functions_to_the_dance_steps_between_psychotherapist_and_client_Phenomenology_and_aesthetics_of_contact_in_the_psychotherapeutic_field.

Spagnuolo Lobb, M. (2018). Aesthetic relational knowledge of the field: A revised concept of awareness in gestalt therapy and contemporary psychiatry. *Gestalt Review, 22*(1), 50–68. https://doi.org/10.5325/gestaltreview.22.1.0050

Spagnuolo Lobb, M. (2020). Dialogues on psychotherapy at the time of coronavirus: An introduction. *Humanistic Psychologist, 48*(4), 340–346. https://doi.org/10.1037/hum0000210

Spagnuolo Lobb, M., & Caccamo, J. (2013). The now-for-next in group psychotherapy: The magic of staying together. *Cahiers de Gestalt-therapy, 2*, 25–38. https://doi.org/10.3917/cges.ns01.0025

Spitz, R. A. (1945). Hospitalism: An inquiry into the genesis of psychiatric conditions in early childhood. *Psychoanalytic Study of the Child, 1*(1), 53–74. https://doi.org/10.1080/00797308.1945.11823126

Staemmler, F. (2006). A Babylonian confusion?: On the uses and meanings of the term 'field'. *British Gestalt Journal, 15*(2), 64–83.

Stern, D. N. (2010). *Forms of vitality: Exploring dynamic experience in psychology, the arts, psychotherapy, and development*. Oxford University Press.

Stolorow, R. D. (2002). Impasse, affectivity, and intersubjective systems. *The Psychoanalytic Review, 89*(3), 329–337. https://doi.org/10.1521/prev.89.3.329.22075

Stolorow, R. D. (2008). The contextuality and existentiality of emotional trauma. *Psychoanalytic Dialogues, 18*(1), 113–123. https://doi.org/10.1080/1048188070 1790133

Stolorow, R. D. (2013). Intersubjective-systems theory: A phenomenological-contextualist psychoanalytic perspective. *Psychoanalytic Dialogues, 23*(4), 383–389. https://doi.org/10.1080/10481885.2013.810486

Stolorow, R. D., & Atwood, G. E. (1996). The intersubjective perspective. *Psychoanalytic Review, 83*(2), 181–194.

Stolorow, R. D., Brandchaft, B., & Atwood, G. E. (1987). *Psychoanalytic treatment: An intersubjective approach.* Analytic Press.

Summers, F. (1994). *Object relations theories and psychopathology: A comprehensive text.* Analytic Press.

Wheeler, M. (2011, October 12). *Martin Heidegger. Stanford Encyclopedia of Philosophy.* https://plato.stanford.edu/entries/heidegger/.

Wulf, R. (1996). *The historical roots of gestalt therapy theory.* Gestalt News and Notes. www.gestalt.org/wulf.htm.

Yalom, I. D. (1995). *The theory and practice of group psychotherapy.* Basic Books.

Yontef, G. (2002). The relational attitude in gestalt therapy theory and practice. *International Gestalt Journal, 25*(1), 15–34.

Yontef, G., & Fuhr, R. (2005). Gestalt therapy theory of change. In A. L. Woldt & S. M. Toman (Eds.), *Gestalt therapy: History, theory, and practice* (pp. 81–100). SAGE.

Yontef, G., & Jacobs, L. (2005). Gestalt therapy. In R. J. Corsini & D. Wedding (Eds.), *Current psychotherapies:* (pp. 299–336). Thomson/Brooks/Cole.

Yontef, G. M. (1993). *Awareness, dialogue & process: Essays on gestalt therapy.* Gestalt Journal Press.

Yontef, G. M., & Simkin, J. S. (1989). Gestalt therapy. In R. J. Corsini & D. Wedding (Eds.), *Current psychotherapies* (pp. 323–361). Peacock.

Zinker, J. (1991). Creative process in gestalt therapy: The therapist as artist. *Gestalt Journal, 14*(2), 71–88.

Chapter 3

Relationality and Indian Culture

Survivors

My first experience in group therapy was more than two decades ago when I was asked by my trainer and head of the center I worked at, to join a group they were conducting for survivors of childhood trauma. I don't recollect the leader communicating to us the exact purpose of the group and from what I remember, I had joined the group because I worked for them and did not want to offend them. From what I understood, the leader was doing some research on the efficacy of group therapy for survivors, but we were not aware of the details. The participants were either working in the organization or were in individual therapy with the leader. Thinking about it now, in retrospect, I believe I would not have joined the group if I had the ability to say 'no' to an elder/authority figure at that time in my life. I had been in individual therapy for almost two years and had participated in quite a few training, therapy and marathon retreat groups. I think I had reached a space where I needed to reflect and assimilate all that I had learned about myself through these therapeutic experiences. As is the case with retrovision, this experience is accompanied with good memories, meaningful learning, nostalgia and poignant regrets.

The survivors group met weekly and we were given some reflective activities and reading to build awareness on what we thought and felt about our experiences and how it had impacted our lives. The group created a safe healing space in the relationship we forged with each other, based on the universality of our shared experiences. I don't recollect the details of how, but I remember that the group disbanded without much ado after a few sessions.

When I started writing this book, I reflectively revisited this experience, from my subjective window, into that time and space. I sat at my desk, visualizing the distant past, feeling fondness for the other members and group leader, a twinge of sadness mixed with thoughtfulness about my experiences and learning. I imagined that room, where we used to meet weekly, watching my peers and me, in our mid-twenties and early thirties, sitting in a circle of nebulous safety: apprehensive, making limited eye contact, nervous smiles, body stooped in shame and with mixed feelings toward the leader. The

DOI: 10.4324/9781003348337-4

support of the circle made up for our individual terrors. We always made it to the sessions on time; we were all compliant to a fault and never questioned, challenged or left the group. The group leader did their best to be empathic and sensitive to our respective narratives.

When we were urged to do some Gestalt experiments like empty chairs, dramatic exaggerations or regressing to the time of the event—asked to scream, kick our perpetrators, most of us chose what was least threatening for us. I personally abstained from talking to an imaginary parental figure for not offering protection. Kicking and screaming was way beyond my comprehension, comfort and tolerance. I stuck to doing the activities that I felt were least threatening to me like sharing my experience with a restrained austerity, listening to the perspectives of the leader and peers and feeling comforted by their empathy. The group leader was sensitive enough not to push, and perhaps I think I have this obdurate impassive presence that blocks external forces. The leader did seem to push the one who complied the most.

What some of us did was passively subvert the hierarchy by politely declining to do the threatening activities. You can call this, 'civil disobedience', 'non-compliance to treatment' or 'ability to regulate one's boundaries'—depending on the cultural-psychological lens with which you look at this behavior. Other than one member, none of the others engaged in the enactments that involved screaming and kicking. At that time, I was not aware of anything discrepant in privately sharing with each other our discomfort and abstaining from directly addressing the discomfiture with the group leader. The group leader probably did not observe these reactions, or given the fact that they were a child of colonial education, may not have been attentive to some of the cultural factors that came in the way of forming the therapeutic relationship. In addition, a rationale for this specific group, structure, frame, timelines and methodology was missing. There was a lack of preparation for what awaited us and a dialogic engagement between the participants and leader to understand how we impacted each other.

The palpable hierarchy between participants and leader, power distance, religious differences and reticence in emotional expression perchance kept us isolated from the leader. These experiences remained inaccessible to us, because we did not engage in reflecting on or talking about it and maintained a silence that probably festered shame. The unexplored civil disobedience movement that stemmed from our own cultural ethos as middle-class Indian women did not portend well for best outcomes. Neither we nor the leader, perhaps, gained the full benefit of the healing powers of human connections and group because we did not discover the possibilities of the dialogic existentialism of Buber's 'inclusion, presence and commitment to dialogue'.

As a group leader now, with a strong relational paradigm, I see some areas for improvement for leading this group that may have facilitated better outcomes. A basic one would have been clear and transparent communications to the members about the purpose, structure, timelines, methodology and the limitations of confidentiality. It would have fostered a feeling of safety if informed and written consent were taken in the eventuality of this being used for research purposes. A concerted focus on the relationship between leader and group members may have opened up opportunities for improving the safety, trust and healing power of relationships. In addition, the process and outcome of this group may have been better if the group leader had been mindful of the immediacy of cultural factors that can impact the alliance and outcome. There were certain unique cultural characteristics like hierarchy, collectivism (in-group collectivism), patriarchy, gender, religion, caste and class that defined how each of us responded in this group. Recognition, exploration, reflection and acknowledgment of these characteristics would have probably helped strengthen the relationship, and within this setting the group therapy could have proven to be more effective. Ongoing dialogue would have helped identify and address possible impasses and ruptures that may have facilitated better outcomes for the group members—especially those related to cultural factors like fear of offending an authority figure.

Relevance of Culture Sensitivity

During the 1950s, there was strong emphasis on the assimilation of the indigenous culture into the dominant culture; by the 1970s there was a shift toward recognizing an ethnic-minority perspective; by the 1980s and 1990s theoreticians and academicians from different fields started advocating for more emphasis on respecting human differences (Kohli, Huber, & Faul, 2010). The multicultural movement that began more than four decades ago was based on observations by theoreticians and practitioners that clients from different minority cultures received poor mental health care. While summarizing significant theoreticians in this field, I agree that psychotherapy practiced with individuals, made to suit a European or American culture, cannot be superimposed on other cultures without taking into account their unique sociocultural environment (Chan, 2003; Chang & Berk, 2009; Chu & Sue, 2011; Gaffney, 2010; Laungani, 2005; Sue & Sue, 1999; Sue & Sue, 1977). Psychotherapists with extensive work experience in Western and Eastern cultural contexts encourage research, training and practice that delves into the cultural differences to bridge the gap between the Western and Eastern ways of thinking. Counseling and psychotherapy are recognized as representing European and American culture, and because it has evolved in the West, it is influenced by Western values and belief systems about what constitutes appropriate human behavior and mental health. These systems may not be applicable to all the multiple cultures that inhabit this world, and a lack of awareness about the cultural factors can become a barrier in effective practice—a barrier counselors need to be mindful of (Arulmani, 2007; Chandras, Chandras, & DeLambo, 2013; Laungani, 2005; Leong & Ponterotto, 2003; Leung, 2003; Leung & Chen, 2009; Rechtman, 2006).

Complexity of Defining Indianness

I have wondered why I used to feel bewildered every time I was asked to look at culture in the context of what I write about psychotherapy practice in India. And probably this is the first time I am consciously engaged in exploring and explaining with this level of seriousness, the importance of taking cultural characteristics into consideration in the practice of psychotherapy, especially group therapy in India. There were many factors that made me wary of talking about Indian culture while writing about the practice of group therapy. As the renowned Indian poet, A.K. Ramanujan (1989) commented in his famous essay more than two decades ago—and it still holds true today—there is no single Indian way of thinking. There are small, and big Indian traditions, ancient and modern, rural, urban and tribal, classical and folk. There are substantial linguistic, religious, caste, regional and cultural diversity in India with notable differences. There are 22 languages recognized by the Indian constitution and each language has its subdialects, and there are nine religions, a caste system and different regions, each with its unique cultural identity and its own special worldview. This makes it unfeasible to talk about a uniform Indian culture or identity, and this is apparent in Ramanujan's writing itself. He talks extensively about the diversity in Indian culture and ironically, he does not bring up the diversity in religions and subsumes Indian society into a Vedic Hindu philosophy. I think the dominance of Hindu philosophy should not be confused with the absence of other philosophies.

Ancient Indian culture has undergone constant changes through migration, invasion, adaptation, conversion, construction, deconstruction and reconstruction that happened due to encounters with other cultures with the advent of Aryans, Muslims, Christian missionaries and European colonialism (Asif, 2020; Chhokar et al., 2007; Kakar, 1978/2012; Kakar & Kakar, 2007; Thapar, 2014). These interactions with other civilizations have touched and brought changes to literature, language, religion, architecture, cuisine, cinema, art and education. Historically, India has had and continues to have a spectrum of democratic, nationalist, right-wing, communist and pockets of military dictatorship with diametrically opposite political allegiances across the country. Moreover, in the last two decades, technology and globalization has had a momentous impact on the cultural characteristics of India, creating a chaotic transitional phase between 'modern' lifestyles on the one hand and traditional values and customs on the other (Bhargava, Gupta, & Kumar, 2016; Gogineni et al., 2018). These cumulative changes over many centuries and the contemporary shifts that are occurring at a far quicker pace have made it all the more difficult to define Indian culture under one singular narrative.

Multiple studies in the field of psychology focusing on cultural shifts taking place in the last two decades seem to point toward a trajectory of cultural transition and confusion that most Indians are going through (Abbassi & Singh, 2006; Kasturirangan, Krishnan, & Riger, 2004; Poulsen, 2009).

These studies reveal how Indians are caught between traditional views about self, family and relationships, and Western education and exposure to media that encourage emancipation and individual well-being. These changes over many centuries and the present changes that are happening at a quicker pace have made it all the more difficult to define Indian culture under one singular narrative. Moreover, the way our history and culture have continued to get shaped and disseminated has profoundly influenced the way we define our identities in the present.

Documented history shows how culture in the Indian subcontinent has changed over time due to exposure to other cultures and religions. For an in-depth understanding of how Indian history was shaped, how culture was represented, what voices were recorded and what voices were silenced, one must read Romila Thapar's (2014) watershed book on Indian history. She is considered the mother of Indian history with a distinguished career spanning more than three decades in writing, teaching and speaking about India's past. She is renowned for her dedicated ability to engage in systematic analysis of historical information, rigorous scholarship, knowledge of decades of engagement in her subject and a definitive political position from which she talks about Indian history and culture.

Thapar has been critical of a communal interpretation of history that claims a uniform Aryan culture that subsumes all other cultures under a single religious Hindu identity. I agree with her that a communal interpretation projects a certain illusory global characteristic of Indianness while in reality there are nuanced characteristics of complex microcultures in India. Through the 19 essays in her book written over the span of Thapar's eminent career as a historical scholar and researcher, a curious reader will discover that the essays cover themes and ask blunt questions pertaining to the current sociopolitical discourse in the country that hugely impact cultural identity. In many of the essays, she ardently invites the reader to ponder whether India's past was only a 'Hindu past' or an expansive plural one, including manifold identities, cultures and religions. She goes on to say that women, scheduled castes and tribes are the survivors of the core values of Aryan civilization in the sense of imbibed slavery and subservience to patriarchal values. One unifying thread that she talks about that cut through Indian history and culture is the disturbing and palpable presence of hierarchy and patriarchy.

Thapar (2014) makes a clear distinction between authenticity of historical events that has to be scrutinized through minute analysis of the evidence, as opposed to unsubstantiated interpretations based on ideology. I agree with her when she says that 'the claims frequently made by groups today to authentic, indigenous identities, unchanging and eternal, pose immense problems for historians' (2014, p. 14). This poses a problem for therapists, too, whether we work with individuals or groups, as it runs the risk of a myopic view of cultural identities. An understanding about the transformational fluidity of identities is important for one's capacity to adapt to change, and holding on to the idea of a singular unchanging identity suggests struggles with adaptation. Often clients come to us with distress because their patterns of responding to the environment have become rigid and are no longer working for them in their relationships. If we look at this psychologically, we know that the ability to become aware of one's patterns, to understand differences with others, and fluidity to experiment with new ways of relating support growth and change.

Identities are never unchanging nor singular because there are multiple identities that emerge from a shared culture and they continue to change over time as the sociopolitical situation changes. Although valuable contributions are being made to find a better understanding of Indian culture and psychology (Rao, 2010; Rao, Paranjpaye & Dalal, 2008), I find it concerning that the available literature explicating Indian psychology is largely Hindu philosophical in its presentations to describe Indian identity, philosophy and psychology. If I talked about Indian culture in a similar vein, then I would reiterate what has already been extensively written about 'Indian philosophy' and 'Indian psychology', and significantly, I would go against my personal values of equity. Given the range and complexity of culture in India, it is not easy to find manifestations of 'Indian' culture that are common to the entire country without exception. Yet practitioners, theoreticians and academicians have attempted to offer a map of the cultural characteristics of Indians to augment an understanding that can support therapists who work with a diverse population (Akhtar & Tummala-Narra, 2005; Arulmani, 2007; Chhokar et al., 2007; Javidan & Dastmalchian, 2009; Hofstede, Hofstede, & Minkov, 2010; Roland, 2005; Kakar, 1978/2012; Kakar & Kakar, 2007; Laungani, 2005). They have attempted to offer a map of the cultural characteristics of Indians to promote an understanding that can support the work of therapists who work with not just Indian clients but probably many Asian, South American, European and Arabic cultures that are marked by collectivism and hierarchies. Practitioners, based on their practical experiences, say that Indians place greater emphasis on feelings and emotions than Westerners; they look for active involvement from their therapists, a deeper connection as opposed to distance, and some may look more for advice and suggestions than self-exploration.

Pittu Laungani (2005), an Indian psychologist with exposure to both Indian and Western culture, wrote extensively on cross-cultural psychotherapy. He argued that the proliferation of multiple theories in the West and their application to Indian culture were detrimental for the building of multicultural counseling bridges. He offered a model that synthesized Indian and Western approaches based on the cultural differences between the two. His model suggests that the multicultural counseling bridge rests on eight pillars of Western and Eastern culture that he has assembled from their respective philosophies. He defines these as: individualism and communalism, cognition and emotionality, free will and determinism, and materialism and spiritualism. He explains the cultural differences between East and West and argues for a synthesis of the two, while appreciating the cultural context and epistemology from which therapists work. He argues that reason and logic do not help us arrive at truth, while also stating that subjective epistemologies have little relevance in promoting objective knowledge. He reiterates that most counseling theories inhabit the world of subjectivity and that it needs to go through rigorous testing to gain objectivity.

Laungani has provided some valuable insights into the cultural characteristics in his model and the importance of understanding this in our work with Indian clients. I agree with him on the importance of being mindful about the eight pillars in our work and the influence of our culture on our practice. However, I was perplexed by what seemed to me a kind of ambivalence about where he stood regarding whether human experiences can be studied objectively or not. On the one hand, he seems to argue that psychotherapy relies too much on rationality, without understanding subjective experiences and differing worldviews, which is antithetical to the Indian cultural ethos. On the other hand, he advocates a scientific temperament and objective knowledge in research and practice of psychotherapy.

I see a paradigmatic conundrum here. It is humanly impossible to locate objective knowledge in the realm of human existence, meaning-making process and behavior. We do not inhabit a clearly defined scientific temperamental space that is free of subjectivity. In fact, the subject we choose to study, write about or research in itself is an act of our subjectivity. It seems to me that the struggle to navigate and accept his Indianness in an alien culture appears to be palpable in Laungani's writing. The dilemma we face when these unbridgeable differences have to be lived with can be quite challenging. I believe that as therapists we have to grapple with these struggles with our 'self', clients and the diverse world we are in a relationship with and make meaning of the ambiguities as far as possible.

Mapping Indian Culture.

Some of the characteristics related to Indian culture, mapped by researchers on national and organizational culture, as well as practitioners and researchers working in a multicultural setting (Boopathi, 2014; Gaffney, 2010, Javidan & Dastmalchian, 2009; Marwah, 2003) have commonalities. Both Hofstede (2011) and the Global Leadership and Organizational Behavior Effectiveness (GLOBE) study have proposed certain cultural dimensions that differentiate Western and Eastern culture like power distance, uncertainty avoidance, individualism versus collectivism, humane orientation and gender egalitarianism. According to Gaffney, in the postcolonial world, many of the countries that were colonies of European imperialism are still struggling to emerge from years of submission. He says that many of us who are in any way representative of a form of dominance—be it racial, political, historical, gender, linguistic or other—have to be aware and sensitive to how this may affect our cross-cultural relations.

While talking about Hofstede's five dimensions of culture, Gaffney (2010) talks also about one of Hofstede's recent dimensions of familism. In individualism, identity is self-defined and interpersonally defined and membership is usually voluntary (United States, United Kingdom, Australia and parts of northern Europe). In familism, identity is defined by family membership, status, hierarchy and responsibilities (Jewish, Arab cultures, Mediterranean area and Asian cultures). In collectivism, identity is in group membership, which is a given, and the group is embedded in the larger social collective (Japan, Korea, China). Gaffney explains further the concept of embedded familism where the family is embedded in other social structures (clan, tribe, ethnic group), which are in turn embedded in the collective of an ethnic group in a defined geographical area, or the family is embedded in segregated social strata (west, south and east Africa, China, India). I find his concept of embedded familism quite relevant to the Indian context, wherein the family is embedded in other social structures, for example, clan and tribe, which are in turn embedded in the collective of an ethnic group within a defined geographical area, or the family is embedded in a segregated social stratum. His extensive work is useful for us to keep in mind while working with Indians; otherwise, we are likely to subsume Indian culture into a larger national culture, whereas there are unique characteristics of ethnic and minority cultures that are embedded in class, caste and religion.

Seminal contributions to understanding aspects of 'Indian' culture (similar to research findings of GLOBE) and how it manifests in psychotherapy have been made by psychoanalysts Kakar (1978/2012) and Akhtar (2005). Research findings and practitioner experiences point toward a higher prevalence of hierarchy, collectivism (in-group and out-groups), humane orientation and gender differentiation in Indian culture. GLOBE scores have ranked India as the second most gender-differentiated country and the second highest on in-group collectivism. Countries scoring high on these cultural practices, such as Iran, India and China, are largely collectivistic and patriarchal societies where cultural memberships regulate treatment of members in groups. Yet there are confounding presentations like the intermediate score for individualism for Indians, which I think has important implications. The individualistic aspect could be due to the dominant Hindu philosophy that holds the individual 'karmically' responsible for the way they lead their lives. It could also suggest the changes taking place in Indian society due to globalization, which are quite far reaching and drastic. In addition, Gaffney's concept of embedded familism offers us a deeper understanding about these variations. Moreover, I believe these variations in research findings are also an invitation for us as therapists to exercise flexibility for the uniqueness of individuals who cannot be easily put into boxes. Individualism and collectivism are a continuum, and I think Indians possess both in differing degrees—the exodus of millions of Indian migrant workers during the pandemic gives us an understanding of this. When the government declared an overnight lockdown and migrant workers were left stranded without jobs, food and transportation and were dying of hunger, they exercised their freedom to walk thousands of miles to arrive back to their homes. I was pained by the news and yet wondered about how they took 'karma' into their own hands using their free will.

The variations in these cultural characteristics that actually presents itself in clinical practice is so mystifying that a preset theoretical framework can prove problematic. Paradoxically, it's important for us to have a theoretical framework for a deeper understanding of the society and culture from which our clients come, to be able to provide sensitive service. This knowledge can inform our professional practice as therapists while working with Indian clients within a group or individual setting. Therefore, I attempt to put forward some characteristics that are based on practitioner experiences, research findings and my knowledge and practice experiences. Given the complexity of defining a singular Indian identity and my pellucid stance about the difference between the words 'Hindu' and 'Indian', I hope to avoid dominant religious or philosophical connotations in how I present these characteristics. The general characteristics common to Indian culture that stand out are illuminated below under the themes of Collectivism, Hierarchy, Gender Disparity, Emotional Restraint and Relationality. I want to reiterate my stance here that generalizations are helpful to give us a working knowledge, and they offer us a map for our practice; however, we cannot afford to rigidly adhere to these because a map does not fully capture the vicissitudes of nature and its tricky terrain.

Collectivism

Unlike the distinctive and individualistic identity of Western selfhood, the core Indian psyche is greatly influenced by the collectivistic nature of Indian society. Within this context, the boundaries between 'self' and 'other' can be indistinct, and often the individual 'I' can get subsumed into a collective 'we'. Kakar (1978/2012) points out the collectivistic nature of Indian society where individualism and independence are not a cherished value in the family system. Making sacrifices for one's family and thinking of the larger good are encouraged. A related feature is the in-group collectivism that shows a tendency in the members to be loyal toward one's own group, friend circle or family, and this makes collaboration with outer groups a challenge. This stems from the joint family system that continues to be common in most parts of India. Izzat (family honor/dignity) is paramount and members are strictly discouraged from taking family secrets outside the system.

Kakar and Kakar (2007), referring to GLOBE study findings, talk about leadership style in organizational settings, where leaders tend to be benevolent and authoritative, willing to be a guide and mentor. Subordinates tend to be highly loyal and willing to stretch the extra mile for approval and validation, thus sustaining an ancient guru–chela (master–disciple) tradition.

Kakar (1978/2012) says that this manifests in the analyst–analysand relationship wherein the analyst is seen as a wise, protective authority figure who is a guide to the analysand, who looks for validation from the analyst. Akhtar and Tummala-Narra (2005) have explained the complications that crop up in psychoanalytic practice stemming from the prevailing collective orientation. A classical neutral stance does not work well with Indian clients, who look for deeper engagement and proximal connections from the therapist. Commenting on the collectivistic nature, they say that Indians look for inter-relational support, which is encouraged and rewarded.

I have experienced some of these characteristics in groups I have facilitated where group members look at me as an idealized or feared authority figure who will be benevolent, protective and guiding. Group members tend to adhere to socially appropriate behaviors and obey authority figures. If there are disagreements, it is likely to get talked about between members, or an in-group can form to vent one's frustrations, thus refraining from addressing this directly with the person concerned. This can create an intangible wall between the leader and group members. I have found that being observant of these cultural factors and engaging in a dialogue regarding these factors with participants may not mitigate the problems completely but it is still useful as a step toward collaborative work.

In many of the groups I have facilitated, I have found some emerging changes. The older generation (people above 40) often show some of the characteristics of the traditional Indian culture described above. However, the younger generation (people in their 20s and 30s) are in a state of flux and there is a higher need for personal autonomy among them accompanied with some anxieties of being rejected for expressing this need. I agree with Kakar (2020) that although individualism has been on the rise since the 1970s, speeded by globalization, it's still negotiated with careful compliance within the family system rather than through open revolt.

In a process-oriented training group I facilitated recently, the cultural differences between the older adults and the younger ones were fairly apparent. At the same time, the younger members' anxiety and fear around individuation were also palpable. Most of the younger adults in the group, who were in their twenties, expressed their frustrations about staying at home, recurrent conflicts with their parents and a desire to leave home. Sita, a woman in her late forties, would make comments about the younger members, who in her experience were 'selfish' for wanting to leave home,

> you don't know how much your parents have suffered and sacrificed to raise you and you have had an easy life [...] now that you are old you are only concerned about leaving them [...] this generation is so selfish.

I was concerned about how this impacted the individual members as well as the group, and explored with Sita and other members their experiences of yearning for independence from their families in their youth. Sita shared memories of her longing for freedom and the frustrations of dealing with her parents, and she also shared her present experiences of anxiety around her adult children wanting to leave home. I encouraged the younger adults in the group to talk about their experiences in their families when they expressed their need to move away, and how these experiences impacted their sense of safety in this group that largely comprised older adults. These process-based explorations can often lead to building awareness into one's internalized beliefs as well as guilt associated with expressing 'self' needs. Considering these aspects from a mental health perspective, the handicap of not having enough opportunities to understand oneself and expectations of focusing largely on others, creates socio-emotional vulnerabilities that predispose individuals to mental health difficulties and interpersonal challenges. At the same time, focusing completely on one's own needs at the cost of others' creates conflicts within oneself and with others.

Hierarchy

Another decisive and rigidly adhered to characteristic of Indian culture is the hierarchical structure that is present across religion, caste, region, gender and ethnicity. The roots of hierarchy can be traced back to patriarchy and the caste system that originated in India thousands of years ago, which imposed a ranked rigidity between the members of its society. The impermeability of this system has sustained a structure of power and powerlessness between its members. A person's self-worth is exclusively determined by the position they hold in the hierarchy of social order, leading to power distance, where people are separated by authority, prestige, power and position in the social system. Kakar & Kakar (2007) dryly observe that Indians are 'perhaps the world's most undemocratic people, living in the largest democracy' (p. 8). They go on to expand this by saying that Indians look at another Indian through the lens of position in the social system, aimed at answering the question, whether the person is superior or inferior to them. Treatment then of the other can be with obsequiousness or arrogant dismissal. I have come across this often in my personal and professional interactions where people providing supportive services (staff members) are treated with abject insensitivity because they are perceived as a 'servant', while a doctor is revered and unchallenged even if they are being remarkably insufferable.

The Hindu caste system is an intricate social system where social roles like one's profession become an inheritance into which one is born and from which there is no escape until death. It is divided into Brahmins (priests/intellectuals/teachers), Kshatriyas (warriors/rulers), Vaishyas (merchants/traders), and Shudras (laborers). Outside of this system are the people who were referred to as 'Achhoots' (untouchables—people who were forced by birth to engage in 'menial' tasks that were considered to be polluting) and renamed as Dalits (meaning the oppressed/broken). Although, constitutionally, the caste system was abolished in 1950, it continues to be deeply embedded in Indian psyche, culture, politics and economic practice. The scheduled caste and tribes continue to be discriminated against and their identities are rarely talked about in the common discourse. Kakar (1978/ 2012) says that the 'principle embodied in the caste system has also put its stamp on the social practices of other religions such as Islam, Christianity and Sikhism which have greater claims to egalitarianism' (p. 28). Among Christians and Muslims there is a hierarchical order based on whether indigenous people who converted were from the lower or upper castes of Hindus.

The hierarchical patriarchal system regulates the Indian joint family structure and continues to be practiced in villages, small cities and urban areas. The patriarch and elders in the family are treated with obedience, filial reverence and silent acquiescence, and this behavior is considered virtuous. Questioning, challenging or expressing one's autonomous views are generally met with disapproval and shaming. The 'elder', 'patriarch', 'leader', 'guru' and the hierarchically subordinate create and sustain a relationship that is marked by personal attachment accompanied by an idealization of and subservience to the superior. Kakar (1978/2012) says that this narcissistic need for an idealized figure may be a universal tendency; however, in India this is also a widespread psychological and tangible social reality where religious and political leaders are worshiped. This percolates into organizations, educational settings, doctor–patient relationships and group therapy settings. A strong preference is shown for an authoritative leader who is strict and nurturing—the proverbial paternal head of the family, who impartially settles disputes, offers protection from the 'other' and maintains in-group cohesiveness. Therapists are usually looked up to as a 'guru' who will guide the client on the right path, and clients tend to be compliant. I agree with Kakar (1978/ 2012) that the Indian child learns very early, when to coax, dissent and retreat into silent disobedience.

A profound understanding of how these hierarchies operate across Indian culture and how it has impacted each individual will help us facilitate awareness and engage in a dialogue with our clients toward healing and change. In the vignette 'Survivors' provided at the beginning of the chapter, you can see the resonance of this in how each of us in the group unconsciously played out our creative childhood strategies within the adult group therapy setting without directly challenging the hierarchy. We can assess this as 'adaptive' or 'maladaptive behavior'; however, as a Gestalt therapist, that is not so much of an area of concern for me. Rather, I would be curious to understand how each of us felt doing this, how it forged or disrupted human connections, and how this has had an impact on our relationships.

In my work, with individuals and groups, I have observed that the hierarchical nature is deeply internalized. Both the young as well as the older members are initially reluctant to call me by name or give feedback to me if I have said or done anything that's hurtful or in contradiction to their beliefs. I have to not just seek feedback consciously but also continue to playfully encourage, support and receive the feedback in a non-defensive manner. Although the hierarchy and power distance are difficult to overcome, members are quite welcoming of the openness to talk about it after the initial discomfiture. In fact, this action of struggling to express oneself to an authority figure in itself becomes an experiment in GGT. This in turn facilitates a process of awareness, an exploration of feelings of guilt and shame, thus opening up the possibilities to develop a greater sense of self-confidence and freedom. It also increases the intimacy between group members as they loosen up the ingrained hierarchy and become more equitable with each other within the group.

Gender Disparity

Kakar's contribution to understanding society in India and its influence on the psychological development of boys and girls is valuable for practitioners. He talks about how the boy child is welcomed and pampered in early infancy and childhood, but distanced from maternal love as he grows older. In addition, boys are encouraged to be strong, self-sufficient and to exercise emotional restraint. At times, boys become victims of the rage women feel toward patriarchal subjugation, leading to a narcissistic injury that often impairs adult intimacy. Commenting on the formation of the Indian woman's identity, he states that Indian women are caught between reconciling their traditional ideals of femininity with modern aspirations. According to him, this gets mitigated to some extent by the shared female cathartic informal group spaces women have created. We can see a reflection of this in women's literature, spanning decades, in which they express their anger at the sociocultural structure that's marked by pervasive discriminations of patriarchy—as reflected in ballads, stories, autobiographies, wedding songs and folk songs (Tharu & Lalitha, 1997).

Tharu and Lalitha (1997), in their detailed anthology tracing women's writing in India from 600 bce to the twentieth century, illustrate women's writing from all walks of life—Buddhist nuns, homemakers, courtesans, saints and widows—that gives voice to unheard voices of Indian women in the last two and a half millennia. This is in contrast to Kakar's (1978/2012) claims that a warm mother–daughter relationship filled with love is persistent in early childhood, which leads to Indian women having good self-esteem, and it is during early adolescence when the girl child is trained in her future roles of daughter-in-law and wife. In adolescence, she is conditioned to be an obedient, caring and sacrificing wife, daughter-in-law and mother, and although this challenges the girl's sense of self-esteem, it gets alleviated by the loving bond she has shared with her mother and continues to share with other significant women in her life. In terms of women bonding that alleviates the distress gender conditioning has on girls, Kakar (1978/2012) is fairly right and fairly blinkered.

I agree with Kakar that in India, 'obedience and conformity, self-lessness and self-denial are still the ideals of womanhood' (1978/2012, p. 52); however, I am skeptical of his views that Indian women have high self-esteem because of the abundance of early maternal love. I think he talks about Indian culture through a principally upper middle-class Hindu male lens and engages in some speculative generalizations that seem to be reductionistic. Moreover, the interchangeable use of 'Hindu' and 'Indian' in his writings is a concern, because it has the risk of subsuming less privileged or minority identities under the prevailing dominant identity. This poses a problem not just for Indian practitioners but also has grave implications for therapists from other parts of the world who work with Indians and have read his book (given that his book has been hailed as the best application of psychoanalysis to Indian culture and been translated into 21 languages around the world).

Coming from one of the few surviving matrilineal families in India and having experienced the privileges of being welcomed into the family at birth more than five decades ago, I have experienced this celebration as superficial, and it does not extend to protecting the girl child from gender roles and biases. Probably this polarity in being welcomed and marginalized has sensitized me to the differential treatment meted out to the girl child in India. In my work with Indian women (individuals and groups) coming from different classes, languages, religions and regions, I have encountered a theme of primary woundedness stemming from the discovery that they were not as wanted and desired as their male siblings. This often gets reinforced by the secondary wounds of differential and prejudicial treatment. Although I have not experienced the primary woundedness, I have encountered experiences that have contributed to the secondary wounds. Existing historical evidence of how Indian women were treated in the past and continue to be in the present, women's literature in India that gives voice to their experiences, alarming rates of female feticide in the last few decades, and the increasing number of crimes against women in the present sociopolitical context, do not tie up well with Kakar's theory of a benevolent Indian female childhood and valued womanhood historically nor presently (Thapar, 2014; Tharu & Lalitha, 1997; Spivak, 1981; Sinha, 2016; Punam, 2015).

Probably due to feelings of being undervalued and encouraged to engage in self-sacrifice and further violations of their personal spaces, many Indian women struggle to directly exercise their independence within their families as well as the larger sociocultural systems. Rather, they have to find female groups to articulate their dissent, struggles and victories through folk songs, theater and writing. Guzder and Krishna (2005), while discussing the impact of culture on Indian feminine identity in working with the diaspora of Indian-origin women, argue for being mindful about the risk a purely Western approach can have on establishing an alliance. They reiterate that

Indian feminine identity is shaped within a gendered hierarchy. Although modernity has shifted part of India's reality to a Western orientation, the family remains quintessential to Indian life with its lasting loyalties and reciprocity. They say that the psychoanalytic stance of neutrality presupposes an empathic attentiveness; however, this assumption can be dangerous given the cultural significance of relationality. The authors argue that Indian women are contending with issues related to their self-identity rooted in their feminine identification with ethnic and host culture, while individuating in multicultural spaces. They recommend a psychotherapy process grounded in the lived experience of the subject rather than neutrality because the cultural context requires a more relational stance to build therapeutic alliance; otherwise, the risk of shaming is higher. I agree with the authors here and resonate with their experiences both from a practitioner as well as a minority perspective.

Emotional Restraint

There is a kind of emotional restraint that marks Indians within their family system, particularly when they have to interact with the world outside the system. From childhood, certain emotions are restricted based on age, gender and hierarchy. As seen in the 'Survivor's' story, each of us in the group was compliant overtly and some of us chose to subvert the hierarchy through Gandhian noncompliance. We were subservient to the power the leader wielded and mostly kept our feelings of hurt, anger, discomfort, frustration and fear in check. Each of us shied away from challenging the authority of the leader. If the leader believed it was good for us to work on our issues using certain techniques, then it was not our place to question or express our discomfort. We coped with our feelings, for not being 'met' by the leader, through connecting with our peers and sharing our frustrations and shame in a passive manner. Moreover, even if our shame had a language, neither we nor the leader found a way to give expression to this and make meaning of it for ourselves.

We had limited understanding of our boundaries, and probably the leader had not given it much thought, so each person allowed their boundaries to be transgressed unknowingly. Our need for belongingness, dependency, empathy and reciprocity was met to some extent within the in-group we formed with peers. We responded to the leader with emotional restraint, which unfortunately is not synonymous with awareness, growth and change. One lone member who complied with all the techniques the leader introduced, seemed sadly separated and isolated from the rest of the group. I feel regret when I think of what their experiences may have been like and wonder how isolated they may have actually felt in the group. At that phase in my life, I possessed limited awareness, cultural sensitivity and wisdom to connect with their experiences.

This experience fostered my gravitation toward an approach to group therapy that is primarily humanistic and relational in its orientation. It has taught me to be more sensitive to the nuances of culture and its impact on each individual within the groups I facilitate. While eliciting their relational experiences with me as group leader, I also use experiments that help them reflect on their different cultural memberships (religion, region, caste, class, gender, sexual orientation, age). I have found that reflection on privileges, and disadvantages, voices that are expressed as well as the silenced, helps facilitate awareness into one's emotions and supports the development of a language to express these in a safe environment.

Relationality

Kakar (1978/2012) points out that a key characteristic of Indians is that they are relational in nature and they prefer the pain of too much closeness to suffering the anxieties of isolation that individuation can bring. Indians generally place a high value on connections with others, and the self is defined in relation to the other. There is a focus on belongingness, dependency, empathy and mutuality. Relationships with others are emphasized, while personal autonomy, space and privacy are considered secondary. The search for connectedness with others and authority figures is a palpable theme. Individuality and independence are not behaviors that are cherished or encouraged. This does not suggest that the individual has no sense of agency or a nascent yearning for it. I think it implies a greater need for ongoing mentorship, guidance from others and feelings of vulnerability/isolation when these are missing in a relationship. This yearning for togetherness, although felt by individuals, may be hidden in Western societies where autonomy, privacy and personal boundaries are highly valued. For many of us who have had opportunities to travel and exposure to other cultures, we can see the overt display of the need for personal boundaries in Western countries where a respectful physical distance is maintained in public spaces. In India, it's fairly common for us to see people standing in perplexing proximity to each other in public spaces, airports, train stations and the like, even if there is sufficient space for maintaining distance. It's almost like the concept of physical distance is alien to us.

The balancing point of the polarity of togetherness and isolation is different in different cultures. Where one is more valued, the other has not had the opportunity to fully develop; however, I believe the necessity for finding a balance is an innate human need. This need for relational connections and its power of healing was probably met to an approximation in the 'Survivors' group with each other. With the leader there was a disconnect, stemming from the unbridgeable hierarchy and power distance and perchance the application of certain Western interventions without sufficient exploration and adaptations to suit the cultural context and individual requirements. Since the relationship is far more important, an excessive focus on the technique or tool may have been counterproductive to the envisaged outcome of therapy.

Akhtar and Tummala-Nara (2005) draw attention to the relative absence of enriching developments in psychoanalytic practice in India and its failure to incorporate the relational and intersubjective schools whose focus of interest is the therapeutic relationship. They speak about the richness of the inter-subjective field perspectives, which emphasize the unique constitution of the analyst, patient and their relationship, and wish that it had percolated to the practice scene in India. While arguing for taking into consideration cultural sensitivity, they say that the relational aspects advocated by the intersubjective school of psychoanalysis would be of particular relevance in the Indian cultural context. I clap my proverbial mental hands in agreement with them.

Need for a Relational Approach

Indian society appears to be in a period of chaotic transition toward power equalization and individualism, although these changes have not fully trickled down to the villages. For Indians who have immigrated to the West, or are born in the West, as well as Indians living in the urban areas in India, traditional parameters continue to operate for choosing academic path, career, marital partners, childrearing and family decisions, yet their exposure to Western culture encourages them to be individualistic and practice autonomy in their choices. Things are changing now. Younger generations do not want hierarchy. They wish for a reduction in power distance, and value autonomy. Many Indian women despite education and financial independence continue to struggle in asserting themselves in their relationships. At the same time, they wish to exercise their right as equal citizens. Although adherence to patriarchal norms is deeply entrenched and agency to leave an unfulfilling or abusive relationship is rarely experienced, there seems to be a rising need to exercise their autonomy. They often seek therapy wanting to resolve these opposing forces they experience as they search for a better quality of life and equitable partnerships.

Globalization has given rise to the evolution of a multicultural self, among the urban middle class, with identities of both a traditional and an inclusive self, leading to conflicts. I have often encountered the manifestations of these struggles in my practice working with Indian urban middle-class clients, trainees, students and supervisees. These complex cultural factors are likely to come up and influence our practice as therapists in establishing a therapeutic bond and desired outcome for our work.

According to Arulmani (2007), who is a practicing counselor in Bangalore, India, available therapy services are largely based on Western approaches to psychology, given that India has a history of being a British colony. He has written a comprehensive and meaningful article examining Western and Indian approaches, suggesting a culturally relevant practice that is more holistic. He states that Western psychology has been largely influenced by the Cartesian mind–body divide and a scientific orientation, while going on to add that the postulate that Western psychology is scientific in temperament and studies human beings as mere objects is probably true of the cognitive behavioral school. However, there have been other approaches (like the humanistic school) that have critiqued this position, and in the last few decades some approaches and practices in the West have moved on to a more phenomenological, existential and relational standpoint. These approaches would be far more relevant to Indian culture given its emphasis on phenomenology and relationality.

During the 1950s, the humanistic existential school, to which GT belongs, embraced a phenomenological stance to make meaning of subjective human experience. As the GT approach continued to grow, experiences of the client, perspectivalism, contextualism and relational experiences became an area of deep psychological interest and applicational value in the therapeutic situation (Yontef & Schulz, 2016). This foregrounding of the relational nature of the therapist–client dyad and its criticality also became more apparent in the intersubjective branch of psychoanalysis also. RGT based on a philosophical and ethical commitment to phenomenology, field theory and dialogic existentialism has strongly emphasized man's connection to self, other, community and the universe, and 'being' is seen in relation to the 'other'. Gestalt theory enables dialogue across cultures, while valuing subjective experience and cultural differences. In discussing and collating the experiences of Gestalt practitioners working in different cultures, Bar-Yoseph (2005) explores concerns that are important to many of us who work relationally across the globe. We inhabit a world that is becoming more turbulent, where dialogue has become a fundamental need to support and sustain relationships. I agree with her that Gestalt theory is a bridge across cultures, a bridge that is constructed with the conviction in the right to be different and respected for these differences. Her book offers practitioners rich experiences of working in foreign lands and offers insight on Gestaltists that supports healing wounds that are socially inflicted.

With the recent trends in relational psychotherapy and the intersubjective school within the psychoanalytic tradition, the emphasis on relationality has become quite prominent in the West, given how relationship is a fundamental need of all human beings. Ironically, traditional Indian psychology that is more intuitive, subjective, relational and experience based seemed to have moved toward a scientific orientation using mostly an empirical method in training, research and practice.

Yet we know that it is humanly impossible to locate objective knowledge in the realm of human existence, the meaning-making process and behavior. We do not inhabit a clearly defined scientific temperamental space that is free of subjectivity. I believe that as therapists we have to grapple with the dilemma we face when we encounter unbridgeable differences, struggles with our own identities and those of our clients and the diverse world we are in a relationship with. With an acceptance of our unique identities, tolerance of our differences from the other, and a willingness to engage in a dialogue we may reach an approximation of understanding. However, it will remain an approximation and we will have to endure that space of uncertainty and unknowing of the other. What may be possible is an aware appreciation of the differences and an acceptance that these differences cannot be fully bridged. It may also support us in being mindful of the challenges we face while working in a heterogeneous Indian cultural context that is marked by profoundly differing subjectivities.

References

Abbassi, A., & Singh, R. N. (2006). Assertiveness in marital relationships among Asian Indians in the United States. *Family Journal, 14*(4), 392–399. https://doi.org/10.1177/1066480706290961

Akhtar, S. (Ed.). (2005). *Freud along the Ganges: Psychoanalytic reflections on the people and culture of India.* Other Press.

Akhtar, S., & Tummala-Nara, P. (2005). Psychoanalysis in India. In S. Akhtar (Ed.), *Freud along the Ganges: Psychoanalytic reflections on the people and culture of India* (pp. 3–25). Other Press.

Arulmani, G. (2007). Counselling psychology in India: At the confluence of two traditions. *Applied Psychology: An International Review, 56*(1), 69–82. https://doi.org/10.1111/j.1464-0597.2007.00276.x

Asif, M. A. (2020). *The loss of Hindustan: The invention of India.* Harvard University Press.

Bar-Yoseph, T. L. (Ed.). (2005). *The bridge: Dialogues across cultures.* Gestalt Institute Press.

Bhargava, R., Kumar, N., & Gupta, A. (2016). Indian perspective on psychotherapy: Cultural issues. *Journal of Contemporary Psychotherapy, 47*(2), 95–103. https://doi.org/10.1007/s10879-016-9348-1

Boopathi, S. N. (2014). A detailed comparison of Finland and India through Hofstede & Globe study. *Global Review of Research in Tourism, Hospitality and Leisure Management: An Online International Research Journal, 1*(1), 72–101.

Chan, D. W. (2003). Multicultural considerations in counseling Chinese clients: Introducing the narrative alternative. *Asian Journal of Counseling, 10*(2), 169–192.

Chandras, K. V., Chandras, S. V., & DeLambo, D. A. (2013). *Counseling Asian-American Indians from India: Implications for training multicultural counselors.* American Counseling Association. www.counseling.org/docs/default-source/vistas/counseling-asian-american-indians-from-india---implications-for-training-multicultural-counselors.pdf?sfvrsn=8.

Chang, D. F., & Berk, A. (2009). Making cross-racial therapy work: A phenomenological study of clients' experiences of cross-racial therapy. *Journal of Counseling Psychology, 56*(4), 521–536. https://doi.org/10.1037/a0016905

Chhokar, J. S., Brodbeck, F. C., & House, R. J. (Eds.). (2007). *Culture and leadership across the world: The GLOBE book of in-depth studies of 25 societies.* Psychology Press.

Chu, J. P., & Sue, S. (2011). Asian American mental health: What we know and what we don't know. *Online Readings in Psychology and Culture, 3*(1). https://doi.org/10.9707/2307-0919.1026

Gaffney, Seán. (2010). *Gestalt at work: Integrating life, theory & practice.* (A. Maclean, Ed.). The Gestalt Institute Press.

Gogineni, R. R., Kallivayalil, R. A., Sharma, S., Rataemane, S., & Akhtar, S. (2018). Globalization of culture: Impact on Indian psyche. *Indian Journal of Social Psychiatry, 34*(4), 303–312. www.indjsp.org/article.asp?issn=0971-9962;year=2018;volume=34;issue=4;spage=303;epage=312;aulast=Gogineni;type=0

Guzder, J., & Krishna, M. (2005). Sita-Shakti @ cultural collision: Issues in the psychotherapy of diaspora Indian women. In S. Akhtar (Ed.), *Freud along the Ganges: Psychoanalytic reflections on the people and culture of India* (pp. 205–233). Other Press.

Hofstede, G. (2011). Dimensionalizing cultures: The Hofstede model in context. *Online Readings in Psychology and Culture, 2*(1). https://doi.org/10.9707/2307-0919.1014

Hofstede, G., Hofstede, G. J., & Minkov, M. (2010). *Cultures and organizations: Software of the mind* (3rd ed.). McGraw-Hill.

Javidan, M., & Dastmalchian, A. (2009). Managerial implications of the GLOBE project: A study of 62 societies. *Asia Pacific Journal of Human Resources, 47*(1), 41–58. https://doi.org/10.1177/1038411108099289

Kakar, S. (1978/2012). *The inner world: A psychoanalytic study of childhood and society in India* (4th ed.). Oxford University Press.

Kakar, S., & Kakar, K. (2007). *The Indians: Portrait of a people.* Penguin India.

Kasturirangan, A., Krishnan, S., & Riger, S. (2004). The impact of culture and minority status on women's experience of domestic violence. *Trauma, Violence, & Abuse, 5*(4), 318–332. https://doi.org/10.1177/1524838004269487

Kohli, H. K., Huber, R., & Faul, A. C. (2010). Historical and theoretical development of culturally competent social work practice. *Journal of Teaching in Social Work, 30*(3), 252–271. https://doi.org/10.1080/08841233.2010.499091

Laungani, P. (2005). Building multicultural counselling bridges: The holy grail or a poisoned chalice? *Counselling Psychology Quarterly, 18*(4), 247–259. https://doi.org/10.1080/09515070500435476

Leong, F. T., & Ponterotto, J. G. (2003). A proposal for internationalizing counseling psychology in the United States. *Counseling Psychologist, 31*(4), 381–395. https://doi.org/10.1177/0011000003031004001

Leung, S. A. (2003). A journey worth traveling: Globalization of counseling psychology. *Counseling Psychologist, 31*(4), 412–419. https://doi.org/10.1177/0011000003031004004

Leung, S. A., & Chen, P.-H. (2009). Counseling psychology in Chinese communities in Asia. *Counseling Psychologist, 37*(7), 944–966. https://doi.org/10.1177/0011000009339973

Marwah, S. B. (2003). Culture and counselling: The Indian paradox implications for professional psychology. In U. Vindhya (Ed.), *Psychology in India: Intersecting crossroads* (pp. 95–107). Concept.

Poulsen, S. S. (2009). East Indian families raising ABCD adolescents: Cultural and generational challenges. *Family Journal, 17*(2), 168–174. https://doi.org/10.1177/1066480709332715

Punam, S. (2015). Female foeticide and health status of girl child in Himachal Pradesh: A case study. *International Journal of Information Research and Review, 2*(3), 480–486.

Ramanujan, A. K. (1989). Is there an Indian way of thinking? An informal essay. *Contributions to Indian Sociology, 23*(1), 41–58. https://doi.org/10.1177/0069966 89023001004

Rao, K. (2010). Psychological interventions: From theory to practice. In G. Misra (Ed.), *Psychology in India: Clinical and health psychology* (Vol. 3, pp. 317–359). Pearson Education India.

Rao, K. R., Paranjpe, A. C., & Dalal, A. K. (Eds.). (2008). *Handbook of Indian psychology*. Cambridge University Press India.

Rechtman, R. (2006). Cultural standards, power and subversion in cross-cultural psychotherapy. *Transcultural Psychiatry, 43*(2), 169–180. https://doi.org/10.1177/13634 61506064847

Roland, A. (2005). Between civilizations: Psychoanalytic therapy with Asian North Americans. *Counselling Psychology Quarterly, 18*(4), 287–293. https://doi.org/ 10.1080/09515070500469830

Sinha, S. (2016). *Indian women writing in English: A feminist study*. Atlantic Publishers & Distributors.

Spivak, G. C. (Trans.). (1981). 'Draupadi' by Mahasveta Devi. *Critical Inquiry, 8*(2), 381–402. https://doi.org/10.1086/448160

Sue, D. W., & Sue, D. (1977). Barriers to effective cross-cultural counseling. *Journal of Counseling Psychology, 24*(5), 420–429. https://doi.org/10.1037/0022-0167.24.5.420

Sue, D. W., & Sue, D. (1999). Barriers to effective multicultural counseling and therapy. In *Counseling the culturally different: Theory and practice* (3rd ed., pp. 133–147). J. Wiley & Sons.

Thapar, R. (2014). *The past as present: Forging contemporary identities through history*. Aleph Book Company.

Tharu, S. J., & Lalita, K. (1997). *Women writing in India: 600 B.C. to the present* (3rd ed.). Oxford University Press.

Yontef, G., & Schulz, F. (2016). Dialogue and experiment. *British Gestalt Journal, 25*(1), 9–21.

Chapter 4

Being and Becoming a Relational Therapist

Fundamentally, the essence of the therapist is embedded in the adage *atmagyan*[1] or the aphorism inscribed at the Temple of Apollo at Delphi, *gnōthi seauton*.[2] We cannot be fully present in a relationship until we are present to our 'self'. Conversely our sense of self develops in relation to the 'other' and our environment. This self is an emergent intersubjective complex phenomenon that is transitory and creative, changing with our contextual experiences (Jacobs, 2016; Staemmler, 2016). The extent to which we show our self, vulnerabilities and mutability in the way we connect with others is regulated by our sense of safety in the field. To quote Jacobs,

> I am strongly aware that my sense of self is more open and fluid when I am in situations with others in which there are supports for my capacities, resources, and vulnerabilities. In situations in which I do not sense welcome, I lose touch with my 'best self', and instead draw on a more enfeebled sense of myself. In either case, as my absorption with my environment grows, be it with a person or something other-than-human, evokes the resources, the sense of self that is most relevant to that moment, without conscious attention on my part.
>
> *2016, p. 259*

A human being is constantly in the process of identifying, regulating and creatively adjusting to their needs and iterating them with the needs of the other.

When this fluidity of self gets stuck for long periods of time and when we are not able to meet our needs in relation to our environment, it then creates distress for us and this is what often motivates us to seek therapy. As therapists, our work involves understanding this pain and the vulnerabilities of our clients and ensuring that we provide interventions within a safe space for best possible outcomes. Our ability to grasp our client's sense of self, supports, relation to the other and environment requires a good understanding of our own self, resources of support and how we relate to others. Our primary tool as therapists is our relationship with our self and the field around us.

DOI: 10.4324/9781003348337-5

I believe this necessitates that the therapist practice self-reflectivity in the process of personal and professional development. For improving this process, the psychoanalytic, family systems, and humanistic–existential approaches to psychotherapy support the notion that personal therapy for therapists be an integral part of psychotherapy training.

Although knowledge, skills and competencies are a prerequisite for an effective practitioner, I believe that the empathic presence of the therapist is fundamental to the practice of psychotherapy. The development of a therapeutic bond between client and therapist depends a lot on the presence and 'being' of the therapist. For me this 'being' is the ineffable essence of who we are. This being, or the essence of who we are, continues to grow, change and evolve in the span of our professional career based on the degree to which we engage in building self-awareness and meaningfully adapt to our environment. This process of growth happens through our engagement in understanding self, in terms of personality functioning, values, beliefs, life experiences and sociocultural context. In that sense and existentially speaking, our being is constantly in the process of 'becoming'. The essence of who we are develops and expands after we come into existence. I think that there is no easy path to this process of being and becoming a compassionate, competent and skilled therapist or group leader.

Even with extensive personal work, supervision and knowledge, we are prone to erring in meeting our clients where they are in their lived space. Disruptions, misunderstandings and ruptures are unavoidable parts of the psychotherapy relationship, whether individual or group. In individual therapy we have to be mindful of this in the dyadic relational field between therapist and client. In couples, family and group therapy these ruptures are far more complex, given the number of participants in the field, since ruptures can happen between members, and between therapist and members. How we recognize it when it happens, track the nonverbal cues of our clients, be aware of our own affective, cognitive and behavioral responses—*sammā-sati*[3]—and how well we regulate it is crucial to the work of being a 'good enough' therapist. Our ability to engage in this process and the willingness and humility to invest in an ongoing dialogue both with ourselves and the client is what helps us sustain the bond and work through the ruptures successfully. The being and becoming of the therapist rests on the pillars that build self-awareness— knowledge, personal therapy, supervision and ongoing personal and professional development. And this personal and professional growth is a lifelong process.

Presently, the issue of whether students and trainees or even practicing therapists require personal therapy during their training continues to be an area of disparate views. This is primarily based on the approach, attitude and beliefs of the paradigm upon which each training program operates. However, training based on the stance that therapists should have attained a significant level of psychological maturation, adjustment and personal awareness in order to be able to help another person do the same is supported by most schools (Norcross, 2005).

Psychoanalysis

Freud spent many years analyzing his own dreams to gain insight into himself and he strongly advocated self-analysis for practitioners. The importance of personal therapy in the training of psychoanalysts began when Freud (1964) postulated that personal analysis is the most indisputable part of psycho-analytic training. He said, 'where and how is the poor wretch to acquire the ideal qualification which he will need in this profession? The answer is in an analysis of himself, with which his preparation for his future activity begins' (as cited in Malikiosi-Loizos, 2013, p. 246). Whether it be classical psycho-analysis, object relations, self-psychology or intersubjective theory, the ther-apist or analyst in training is required to engage in some form of therapy to develop self-awareness because, the analyst can only interpret the influence the transference is having on her if she is well aware of her own neurosis and transference, her own internal objects (Parth et al., 2017, p. 194). Just as we evoke certain feelings in clients, they also evoke certain feelings in us— these can be suppressed but cannot be avoided or ignored. If it is outside our awareness and acted out unknowingly, it can cause disruptions, and in the worst-case scenario, it can lead to iatrogenic damage to the client and the outcome of therapy.

I remember one of the interviews I conducted during my doctoral research where I was exploring client experiences with the therapist in psychotherapy in India. In the phenomenological interview, a young adult participant narrated her experience with her therapist who told her that she shouldn't be having all these problems with her parents since she was from an upper-middle-class family. She was advised to be grateful because she was privileged compared to the poor families who do not even have access to food. When the client stopped going to her sessions, the therapist called her multiple times and sent text messages accusing her of being arrogant and disrespectful of the therapist. This is a disturbingly severe example of therapeutic breach. Some level of misunderstanding and rupture cannot be avoided; however, I think self-awareness on the part of the therapist can help navigate the ruptures. Crucially, it can help us understand our countertransference reactions and respond to our clients with care and sensitivity, as opposed to acting out our countertransference with serious consequences to our clients.

Family Systems

The 'being' or 'self of therapist' as systemic therapists call it (Lum, 2002; Reupert, 2006; Timm & Blow, 1999) is a more important factor in the process and outcome of therapy than the orientation or interventions chosen by the therapist. Systemic approaches like experiential family therapy developed by Carl Whitaker, narrative family therapy supported by Michael White, conjoint family therapy of Virginia Satir, and emotion focused family therapy of Sue Johnson stress the importance of self-exploration on the part of trainees, particularly through their participation in group or family therapeutic settings (Malikiosi-Loizos, 2013). For Satir, the ongoing development of the self of the therapist was crucial to becoming an effective therapist. Satir in her residential training programs in family therapy dedicated a lot of time to the experiential training of future family therapists. She believed that therapists need to expand awareness in their family relationships and resolve unfinished family-of-origin issues as part of their own healing. This, she believed, was critical to facilitating, with congruence, the healing of clients' family-of-origin issues. The Satir model encourages a process of awareness into the unfinished past, acceptance of self and the finding of creative ways for relating with the world. Timm and Blow (1999) say that the 'self-of-the-therapist work is a critical component of therapist training and development and that it makes the difference between mediocre and excellent therapists' (p. 333). I do agree that the therapist's personal work is crucial to their training and professional development. This is true of whether we work with individuals, families or larger groups.

In group therapy, the here-and-now interactions of the members and the leader with each other can be reminiscent of certain patterns from family of origin. In a group I conducted in the early years of my practice, Sara would often share an event that was traumatic in her relationship with her family of origin. When group members or I expressed concern and curiosity, she would respond saying she was fine. Her narratives were marked by significant emotional distress and quick recovery when asked how she was feeling. Over ongoing meetings, members in the group and I found this experience frustrating, and in one particular meeting a few of the members expressed their anger at how they experienced her disclosure and abrupt withdrawal. Although I processed how each of them felt and how Sara felt, my focus was on Sara and her pattern of sharing and withdrawing when empathized with. I failed to explore further what could be at the root of responses from the rest of the members and my embodied experience.

It was after that day's meeting and upon self-reflection, followed by consultation with my supervisor, that I became more aware of my way of being in my family of origin as a child and my personal frustrations that can get triggered when emotions of vulnerability are swallowed rather than expressed. I went back to the next meeting with clarity about my own dynamics and a tentative understanding of the dynamics of the other group members. Further exploration in the group and asking about how Sara and other members responded to their families as children helped us own the field that we had co-created. Sara was used to her feelings being ignored and being expected to be strong in her family. It was painful for her to express her anguish. Acknowledgment of this by the group evoked feelings of shame around being vulnerable that would make her withdraw. Most members in the group had similar experiences of expressing painful emotions and withdrawing that they felt ashamed and angry about. The intensity of anger they directed toward Sara came from their own unprocessed anger and shame toward themselves. This led to Sara feeling confused and hurt, thus creating an impasse in the group. My momentary lapse in not making meaning of my irritation affected the way I explored the reactions of each member and added to the hurt and confusion Sara felt. As Jacobs (2009a) says, as therapists we are first and foremost a human being, and we can only attune to our client from the depths of our own subjectivity. I agree with her that both parties contribute to attunement and misattunement and are dialogic partners constrained by their limitations. Without the support I could draw from my personal therapy and supervision, this misattunement would have probably slipped through, and the group and I would have made the Cartesian error of seeing Sara's behavior as the problem rather than looking at it as a co-created event. To connect with each member's experience and humbly express remorse at how Sara may have felt scapegoated was a redeeming experience for us.

Cognitive Behavior Therapy

Classical CBT did not initially mandate personal therapy as part of the training of future therapists. Therapy was believed to be a learning process where therapists taught their clients how to change problematic thoughts, beliefs and maladaptive behaviors using various tools. However, in recent years, this attitude has changed and cognitive-behavioral approaches advocate the importance of personal therapy (Bennett-Levy & Finlay-Jones, 2018; Bennett-Levy, 2019; Gale et al., 2017). Based on recent research and theoretical evidence, the authors hypothesize that the personal and interpersonal qualities of therapists play a key role in client outcomes. They advocate personal practice as the most effective way to achieve therapist development and better client outcomes. Gale et al. (2017) say that the therapist's personal practice of therapy techniques can have a decisive impact on a range of areas, including empathy for the client, therapeutic understanding, therapist skills and self-awareness.

Recent trainings in different forms of CBT draw extensively on personal practice during training, and ongoing personal practice is encouraged for the therapists. Theoreticians and practitioners with a CBT approach recommend mindfulness and meditation-based programs to train therapists in developing therapeutic presence (Bennett-Levy & Finlay-Jones, 2018; Bennett-Levy, 2019; Siegel, 2010). Siegel has been influenced by Zen Buddhism, which has gained popularity in Western psychology over the last three decades. He recommends that therapists bring an awakened mind to focus on things as they are, by being present with what is happening in the here and now. He argues that the therapist's mindfulness and presence—and not the interventions—are the strongest predictor of client improvement. It is heartening for me to see that CBT, which is an important part of psychotherapy training and practice in India, advocates the importance of self-reflection for therapists because it plays a key role in client outcomes. I do agree with Bennet-Levy (2019) that personal practice and self-reflectivity is the most effective way to achieve changes in therapist's personal and interpersonal qualities. They recommend that empirical research should move beyond asking whether or not personal practice is effective, and toward a more sophisticated set of questions like: what kind of personal practice, what is most effective with which practitioners? in what contexts? To further this process, they also advocate that trainers and researchers need to be supported to include personal practices in therapist training and also to undertake research to evaluate their impacts.

Existential–Humanistic School

Now I come to the school that I am closest to in my essence as well as allegiance—the existential-humanistic school, which GT is part of. Existential philosophers like Martin Heidegger, Friedrich Nietzsche, Maurice Merleau-Ponty, Jean-Paul Sartre and Viktor Frankl agreed that existence comes before essence. We are thrown into human existence first and the essence of who we become develops in relation to our environment and the choices we make. The existentialists were in agreement that the human being is dynamic and has the ability to be self-reflective and transform the self through the process of life, and their journey in the world. From the point of view of existential psychotherapy, there are three modes of the world. The first is 'Umwelt', meaning 'world around', which is the biological world; the second is 'Mitwelt', literally the 'with-world', which is the world of one's fellow human beings; the third is 'Eigenwelt', the 'own-world', which is the relationship to one's self (Van Deurzen & Adams, 2011; Krug, 2009; May, 1983; May & Yalom, 1989). The Umwelt is the environment; the Mitwelt is the world of relationships with other human beings; and the Eigenwelt is our internal world and influences—the way in which we relate to the real world. The human being lives in all these three modes of relationships concomitantly. Whether we work with individuals or groups, the client's relationship with self, with fellow human beings and with the environment plays a significant role in his psychological well-being. I believe that as therapists it's important for us to be curious about our client's relationship with self and their environment, which includes how they experience their relationship with us and how that impacts their well-being. Concomitantly, we need to gain a deeper understanding into our relationships with the three modes. To support this process, we need to be in a reflective dialogue with our self to understand our subjective ways of relating to the three modes. This is especially crucial to the group therapy setting, where Umwelt,

Mitwelt and Eigenwelt are constantly interacting, being influenced by, and influencing each other.

Rogers (1995) describes his personal stance on the importance of self-reflection, which informs the practice of humanistic therapy—'It is only when I can be myself, when I can accept myself, that it is possible for me to understand and accept others' (p. 19). Yalom (2002) has emphasized the importance of personal therapy for therapists, underlining its importance in psychotherapy training. He stresses the need for therapists to be familiar with their own dark side and be able to empathize with all human wishes and impulses, especially since this experience permits the student therapist to experience many aspects of the therapeutic process from the patient's seat—the tendency to idealize the therapist, the yearning for dependency, the gratitude toward a caring and attentive listener and the power granted to the therapist. I agree with him when he says that this process is lifelong for therapists and that at different stages of life, they need to seek therapy based on the developmental challenges that one can go through as a human being.

'Being' of Therapist and Gestalt Therapy

For the training of a Gestalt therapist, to practice in a truly relational way that gives primacy to the being and to becoming, personal therapy is a necessary requirement. As therapists we are shaped by our historical and cultural biases, which are unavoidable parts of being in relationship with Umwelt, Mitwelt and Eigenwelt. GT sees the therapist as first and foremost a human being in relation to their own world just as the client is. Wheeler and Axellson (2015), commenting on the training scenario, point out how

> disturbing it is to note that the current trend in training programs for therapists is to have minimal or no requirements for trainees to engage in the therapeutic process as clients. To imagine embarking on that complex work without a deep voyage through one's own history and capacities for contact, complexity, and creativity makes no sense and may in fact be a path toward rigidity or damage to the self and others. Key is the relational stance. Because we build relationships by inquiring deeply into the phenomenology of our client's world (and thereby learning more about our own), we need a strong base of contact capacity ourselves to act as the "holding relationship" for our client's development.
>
> *p. 121*

GT gives serious prominence to self-awareness and is firm on its demand that trainees pursue their personal therapy for a mindful practice of RGT (Clarkson, 2005; Yontef & Jacobs, 2010; Yontef, 2002). This stance presupposes that the therapist can make errors in relating with the client, just as the client can make errors in relating with the therapist. Yontef (2002) says that this kind of therapeutic stance requires the therapist's presence—acknowledging having been wrong, arrogant and mistaken when they have said or done something that the client has experienced as hurtful.

The focus on talking earnestly about the relational aspects of inclusion, presence, and dialogue started in the early 1980s. Buber's philosophy was an invitation for therapists to shun the role of a subject-to-object way of relating and enter the relational field of phenomenology for both (Jacobs, 2009b; Stawman, 2009; Yontef, 2009). This stemmed from a growing insight into how dialogic existentialism was fundamentally a relational viewpoint. However, Yontef (2009) says that it would often get violated by many talking the language of relationality yet failing to walk the talk.

This kind of relational and phenomenological attitude requires awareness, recognition and the bracketing off of the preconceptions that we carry. Staemmler (2010) says that we are shaped by our historical and cultural field, and even if we try to practice some kind of bracketing and become aware of biases in our work, we remain quite far away from a radical 'antiseptic' phenomenological stance. Our attempts will continually remain attempts and our observations will be colored by our subjectivities. He goes on to state that this is not essentially a disaster but a positive aspect of our being as human as our clients. He says that this level of attunement to the self and the other requires humility and awareness on the part of the therapist; otherwise, there is a danger of adopting an attitude of arrogance that unwittingly exerts an autocratic control over the client, thus negating clients' experience.

In GT training, skill and self are seen as fundamental to working as a Gestalt therapist. Therefore, theory, personal and skill development are woven together, which is further supported by ongoing supervision. This system fits with the theory itself, which asserts that the therapeutic significance of an intervention lies in the co-created relationship rather than in the administration of a standard technique (Bar-Yoseph et al., 2008; Yontef & Schulz, 2016). Thus, the Gestalt trainer/therapist must evaluate the implications of any intervention from a theoretical as well as a relational perspective. Bar-Yoseph et al. (2008) and Yontef and Schulz (2016) give examples of how a suggestion for an experiment may lead to an empty enactment by an overcompliant client, rejection by a combative client or interested engagement from a client who is not stuck in either of these poles. The performance of an experiment, or the client following the therapist's suggestions, is not in itself the purpose of the experiment. The purpose lies in the awareness that the experimentation leads to, in terms of new material. For example, the client's ability to say no to the experiment in itself can be an experiment for both the client and the therapist to gain a relational understanding. The therapist must therefore be able to assess the meaning of each intervention in the ongoing flow within the therapeutic relationship.

This level of reflectivity requires a multipronged approach, and I agree with Bar-Yoseph et al. (2008) that 'training, supervision, and personal therapy are the three building blocks in the creation of an ethical, integrity-full, creative and thoughtful practitioner' (p. 131). I believe this profound understanding of the implications of interventions from a theoretical and relational perspective is very useful in general for us as Gestalt therapists. Specifically, from my experience as a group therapist and trainer in India, this is of immense value given the likelihood of many of our clients engaging in an intervention to comply with us. To be able to make meaning of these intricacies in our work requires a relationship with ourselves.

The Training of Therapists

As discussed earlier, many approaches place emphasis on the criteria required for the personal and professional development of the therapist. In Britain, the Division of Counselling Psychology of the British Psychological Society requires that trainees in counseling psychology engage in at least 40 hours of personal therapy or personal development programs (Rizq & Target, 2008). The European Federation of Psychologists' Associations (EFPA) requires at least 100 hours of personal development as specified by different therapeutic schools (Malikiosi-Loizos, 2013). Both individual and personal development groups have been advocated to enhance self-awareness in trainees and practicing therapists as a vehicle for personal and professional insight (Lennie, 2007; Norcross, 2005; Norcross et al., 2008; Pieterse et al., 2013).

The ability to reflect on self occurs in an interpersonal context, whether it be individual or group therapy. In a qualitative study conducted by Myers (2003), the experiences of 16 graduate students enrolled in counselor education that required self-reflection and interpersonal interaction were explored. Through written narratives, participants shared that engaging in activities designed to enhance self-awareness served to promote their professional and personal development. In a group process, interacting with one's peers who face similar struggles and find creative ways to meet the challenges of life and work helped trainees feel supported and connected in their subjective experiences of isolation. Myers (2003) says that for the prospective counselor, facing personal vulnerabilities and allowing others to witness them promotes self-compassion and develops the possibilities for expanding empathic relationships with others. Furthermore, belonging to an ongoing group that is engaged in sharing, inclusion, presence, introspection and mutually challenging interpersonal interactions offers a lived experience to the therapeutic encounter.

The benefits of this method of training that focuses on the acquisition of knowledge, skills, competency and awareness for professional development of the therapist has been supported by many experts in the field (Elton-Wilson, 1994; McLeod, 2003), and by subjective accounts of therapists and trainees in various studies (Grimmer & Tribe, 2001; Kumari, 2011; Rake & Paley, 2009). Barrett-Lennard (1997) describes the limitations of therapists who are aversive to self-reflection and are inattentive to their inner selves, or who anxiously ward off impulses and uncomfortable feelings within the self. He says that they are unlikely to be very receptive to the felt inner experiencing and meanings of others. Therefore, when training programs neglect to process the self of the therapist, there is an implied message and collusion with the therapist trainees to ignore the healing of their own unresolved issues (Shadley, 2000). Whether one works with individual clients or with groups, development of personal and professional awareness needs to be an essential part of a therapist's training.

Leader's Awareness in Group Therapy

Practitioners of group therapy see the group as a space where individuals can become aware of intrapersonal and interpersonal isolation and conflicts and the group can facilitate healing and growth (Cole & Reese, 2017; Fairfield, 2004; Feder, 1980; Feder, 2013; Kepner, 1980; Yalom, 1975). Yalom (1975), postulating from a group therapy perspective, says that clients fall into despair because of their failure to forge and sustain intimate and stable relationships with others. In relation to the 'circle', participants develop awareness into ways of 'self-functioning', ways of relating with others, and ways of significantly taking responsibility for their intrapersonal and interpersonal challenges. Yalom's conceptualization of his role as a therapist is that 'we are all in this together and there is no therapist and no person immune to the inherent tragedies of existence' (Yalom, 2002, p. 8). Yalom's (2002) stance of seeing the self as a 'fellow traveler' finds resonance in the practice of GGT. The GGT leader's obligation to personal and professional growth is essential to the vitality of the group. I agree with Wheeler and Axelsson (2015) that, to imagine embarking on this complex work of being a therapist without engaging in a profound voyage through one's own history and capacities for contact, complexity and creativity makes no sense and may in fact be a path toward rigidity or damage to the self and others. Because we build relationships by inquiring deeply into the phenomenology of our client's world (and thereby learning more about our own), we need a strong base of contact capacity ourselves to act as the 'holding relationship' for our client's development (Wheeler and Axelsson (2015), p. 121). GGT practitioners Cole and Reese (2017) recommend leaders do their own personal work, seek supervision about the groups they run and continue to develop supportive networks that help the leader as well as the group. They go on to emphasize the criticality of a leader's responsibility in creating a safe container for the members while holding, listening and resonating with the members as well as the whole group. The leader holds greater responsibility toward the welfare of the group, to actively listen and track each member's subjective experiences while being attuned to one's own embodied experience. My experiences of being part of process-oriented training groups as well as a group leader leads me to agree with them when they say that this safe space we can create as group leaders allows the group members to develop trust over time and share their emotions, thoughts, feelings and bodily experiences in the group space:

> no matter how much work we have done on ourselves we can never transcend our humaneness, our dark shadows, and the advantage of GT is that it teaches us it's okay to be vulnerable and human, to embrace our humanity, we can only strive to be curious, stay in contact with our vulnerabilities and acknowledge them.
>
> *Cole & Reese, 2017, p. 82*

Recently in one of the training groups that I have been conducting, a member brought up their anger and disappointment with me for not having created enough time for them to express their recent grief related to the loss of a loved one to the pandemic. While sharing this in the group, they also brought up their feeling of injustice that I have given some other members more space and time. Although at that given moment I felt perplexed and blindsided, I parked that for a while and asked them more questions about their experience and listened to their expressions of anger toward me, which was challenging for both of us. While admitting to my remorse at causing pain through my failure to have picked up some of the nonverbal cues from them, I also acknowledged that I can at times miss out on cues of what they may want from me and they can point it out to me when I do so. This does not mean that I would be able to create time or be attuned always to meet their needs but I am open to listening to their disappointments. I think it's useful to keep in mind what Feder (2013) says, while highlighting many responsibilities of the leader in GGT: the most important responsibility of the leader is to create a safe enough space for the group members to do their work.

Challenges in India

Although psychotherapy and counseling as a profession are growing in India, it is still a 'fledgling discipline' (Arulmani, 2007) with challenges to the training of mental health practitioners. The imparting of knowledge and theories primarily based on Western concepts of personality and mental health is fairly comprehensive, while the resources to provide experiential training, personal therapy and individual supervision to practitioners is limited. Manickam (2010) says that psychotherapy training requires supervision of the work of the young therapist by an experienced therapist, yet given the paucity of time and personnel, this crucial part of training often remains truncated. He points out that there is an increased demand from psychotherapy trainers and trainees for better psychotherapy training procedures. However, supervision and personal work are quite neglected for various reasons like shortage of time, impracticality of long-term analysis and a negligent attitude toward the professional development of both training institutes as well as students.

A young therapist in our country often ends up with inadequate intrapersonal and interpersonal awareness, skills and competencies. Although some training organizations, institutions and educational settings encourage and provide supervision to students, utilizing it depends on the time, dedication and personal stance of supervisor and supervisee (Tharyan, 2000). Supervision and personal development for the beginner therapist are either absent or get curtailed in this field condition. Given these disturbing gaps in the training of a therapist in India, I feel disappointed to note that personal therapy remains a distant goal in the professional and personal development of the therapist. At the same time, it's heartening for me that a few of the smaller educational institutions like Parivarthan and Montfort College in Bangalore emphasize both individual and group therapy for their counseling psychology trainee therapists. Christ University in Bangalore has eight hours of mandated therapy as well as process groups for counseling psychology students at the postgraduate level. However, few trainees sustain their personal work beyond the mandated requirements. This could probably be due to personal beliefs about seeking therapy, stigma, systemic problems of finding a good match in therapists, inadequate personnel and financial constraints.

Given the paucity of resources and mental health practitioners, group therapy would be a good option in India for both clients (Easvaradoss & Cabral, 2015; Singhal et al., 2018; Sharma et al., 2017) and trainee students who struggle to access individual therapy. Based on my experience, as well as the last seven decades of Gestalt practitioners/teachers' experiences, GT is a powerful tool to impart training in a group setting (Feder, 1980; Kepner, 1980; *PHG*, 1951; Spagnuolo Lobb, 2019). Although I strongly believe that individual therapy is important for a trainee or veteran practitioner and group therapy cannot be a substitute for it, I also believe that the group is a powerful agent of awareness and growth in individual, group and the larger social context. Given the fact that effective practice as a therapist requires knowledge, skills and self-reflectivity to facilitate awareness in the client, it's imperative for the therapist to engage in this process, not just to gain skills experientially but also to work through some of their own issues and also experience what it feels like to be a client. Many trainees who enter this profession come with their share of fears, anxieties, interpersonal difficulties and concerns about their personal and professional selves. In a process-oriented training group, the members get an opportunity to express their concerns, feel the universality of their anxieties, address some of their family of origin issues and have the opportunity to develop interpersonal skills. As Yalom (1975) says, the most effective way to teach group therapy is to provide the students an opportunity to be involved in some kind of personal group experience. If they are in a group experience where there's a focus on the here and now, and a leader who is attuned to the intrapersonal and interpersonal dynamics, it's a learning experience they will remember, and they will look for ways to make use of that in their practice.

As a Gestalt therapist, trainer and supervisor practicing in Bangalore, India, I have been clear regarding my stance about the need for personal therapy for trainees. All trainees who register for the training are required to be in individual therapy. However, attending group therapy and the annual residential retreats is left to the discretion of the trainees. Given the limited resources, only eight trainees are taken on for the intensive training every two years or so, and the training is experiential with a substantial focus on process work on which the theory of relationality is grounded. I have found this model to be quite useful in the training of the therapists in ensuring that they provide meaningful services to the primary stakeholders. This training and practice that are based on the foundational assumptions of GT, have shown that the therapists develop remarkable sensitivity and competency in sustaining a bond with their clients. In addition, they have been better equipped in facilitating awareness and growth for their clients over the period of their therapeutic work.

The whole rationale for the inclusion of personal development in the training of therapists goes back to the concepts of self-analysis, self-awareness and self-actualization introduced by Freud, and subsequently, existential, humanist, and Gestalt therapists in sync with the ideas of *atmagyan* and *gnōthi seauton*. Trainees must learn to distinguish their emotions and be aware of their beliefs, values, moral principles, sociocultural and political identities, and their reactions to various stressful situations. The pathway to this is for the bravehearted, because journeys of personal awareness are irrevocably linked to our personal woundedness, which is painful. However, if we don't invest in our own *atmagyan*—at an individual level—our fluidity and growth become stuck. At a larger relational level, there is a risk of not being fully present to our clients because we have shied away from being fully present to ourselves.

Notes

1 Sanskrit word meaning 'knowledge of the soul or self'
2 This is an ancient Greek aphorism that means 'Know thyself' and is considered to be Socrates' admonition for introspection.
3 Is a Pali word meaning 'right' mindfulness where one is attentive to one's thoughts, emotions, speech and actions.

References

Arulmani, G. (2007). Counselling psychology in India: At the confluence of two traditions. *Applied Psychology, 56*(1), 69–82. https://doi.org/10.1111/j.1464-0597.2007.00276.x

Baldwin, M. (2000). Interview with Carl Rogers: On the use of the self in therapy. In M. Baldwin (Ed.), *The use of self in therapy* (2nd ed., pp. 29–38). Haworth Press.

Bar-Yoseph, T. L., O'Neill, B., Philippson, P., & Brownell, P. (2008). Training of therapists. In P. Brownell (Ed.), *Handbook for theory, research, and practice in gestalt therapy* (pp. 104–121). Cambridge Scholars Publishing.

Barrett-Lennard, G. T. (1997). The recovery of empathy: Toward others and self. In A. C. Bohart & L. S. Greenberg (Eds.), *Empathy reconsidered: New directions in psychotherapy* (pp. 103–121). American Psychological Association.

Bennett-Levy, J. (2019). Why therapists should walk the talk: The theoretical and empirical case for personal practice in therapist training and professional development. *Journal of Behavior Therapy and Experimental Psychiatry, 62*, 133–145. https://doi.org/10.1016/j.jbtep.2018.08.004

Bennett-Levy, J., & Finlay-Jones, A. (2018). The role of personal practice in therapist skill development: A model to guide therapists, educators, supervisors and researchers. *Cognitive Behaviour Therapy, 47*(3), 185–205. https://doi.org/10.1080/16506073.2018.1434678

Clarkson, P. (2005). *Gestalt counselling in action* (3rd ed.). SAGE.

Cole, P. H., & Reese, D. A. (2017). *New directions in gestalt group therapy: Relational ground, authentic self.* Routledge.

Easvaradoss, V., & Cabral, V. (2015). Impact of cognitive behavior group therapy on the psychological functioning of adolescents from dual earner families. *Indian Journal of Health & Wellbeing, 6*(2), 177–180.

Elton-Wilson, J. (1994). Is there a difference between personal and professional development for a practicing psychologist? *Journal of Educational and Child Psychology, 11*(3), 70–79.

Fairfield, M. A. (2004). Gestalt groups revisited: A phenomenological approach. *Gestalt Review, 8*(3), 336–357. https://doi.org/10.5325/gestaltreview.8.3.0336

Feder, B. (1980). Safety and danger in the gestalt group. In B. Feder & R. Ronall (Eds.), *Beyond the hot seat: Gestalt approaches to group* (pp. 41–52). Brunner/Mazel.

Feder, B. (2013). *Gestalt group therapy: A practical guide.* Create Space Independent Publishing and Ravenwood Press.

Freud, S. (1964). Analysis terminable and interminable. In J. Strachey (Ed.), *The standard edition of the complete psychological works of Sigmund Freud* (Vol. 23, pp. 216–253). Hogarth Press.

Gale, C., Schröder, T., & Gilbert, P. (2017). 'Do you practice what you preach?' A qualitative exploration of therapists' personal practice of compassion focused therapy. *Clinical Psychology & Psychotherapy, 24*(1), 171–185. https://doi.org/10.1002/cpp.1993

Grimmer, A., & Tribe, R. (2001). Counselling psychologists' perceptions of the impact of mandatory personal therapy on professional development: An exploratory study. *Counselling Psychology Quarterly, 14*(4), 287–301. https://doi.org/10.1080/09515070110101469

Jacobs, L. (2009a). Attunement and optimal responsiveness. In L. Jacobs & R. Hycner (Eds.), *Relational approaches in gestalt therapy* (pp. 131–169). Gestalt Press.

Jacobs, L. (2009b). Relationality: Foundational assumptions. In D. Ullman & G. Wheeler (Eds.), *Cocreating the field: Intention and practice in the age of complexity* (pp. 45–72). Gestalt Press.

Jacobs, L. (2016). Meaningfulness, directionality and sense of self. In J.-M. Robine (Ed.), *Self: Une polyphonie de gestalt-thérapeutes contemporains* (pp. 251–260). L'Exprimerie.

Kepner, E. (1980). Gestalt group process. In B. Feder & R. Ronall (Eds.), *Beyond the hot seat: Gestalt approaches to group* (pp. 5–24). Brunner/Mazel.

Krug, O. T. (2009). James Bugental and Irvin Yalom: Two masters of existential therapy cultivate presence in the therapeutic encounter. *Journal of Humanistic Psychology, 49*(3), 329–354. https://doi.org/10.1177/0022167809334001

Kumari, N. (2011). Personal therapy as a mandatory requirement for counselling psychologists in training: A qualitative study of the impact of therapy on trainees' personal and professional development. *Counselling Psychology Quarterly, 24*(3), 211–232. https://doi.org/10.1080/09515070903335000

Lennie, C. (2007). The role of personal development groups in counsellor training: Understanding factors contributing to self-awareness in the personal development group. *British Journal of Guidance & Counselling, 35*(1), 115–129. https://doi.org/10.1080/03069880601106849

Lum, W. (2002). The use of self of the therapist. *Contemporary Family Therapy, 24*(1), 181–197. https://doi.org/https://doi.org/10.1023/A:1014385908625

Malikiosi-Loizos, M. (2013). Personal therapy for future therapists: Reflections on a still debated issue. *European Journal of Counselling Psychology, 2*(1), 33–50. https://doi.org/10.5964/ejcop.v2i1.4

Manickam, L. S. (2010). Psychotherapy in India. *Indian Journal of Psychiatry, 52*(7), 366. https://doi.org/10.4103/0019-5545.69270

May, R. (1983). *The discovery of being: Writings in existential psychology.* W. W. Norton.

May, R., & Yalom, I. D. (1989). Existential psychotherapy. In R. J. Corsini & D. Wedding (Eds.), *Current psychotherapies* (pp. 363–402). F E Peacock.

McLeod, J. (2003). *An introduction to counselling* (3rd ed.). Open University Press.

Myers, S. (2003). Reflections on reflecting: How self-awareness promotes personal growth. *Person-Centered Journal, 10*, 3–22. https://adpca.org/wp-content/uploads/2020/11/10_1_3.pdf.

Norcross, J. C. (2005). The psychotherapist's own psychotherapy: Educating and developing psychologists. *American Psychologist, 60*(8), 840–850. https://doi.org/10.1037/0003-066x.60.8.840

Norcross, J. C., Bike, D. H., Evans, K. L., & Schatz, D. M. (2008). Psychotherapists who abstain from personal therapy: Do they practice what they preach? *Journal of Clinical Psychology, 64*(12), 1368–1376. https://doi.org/10.1002/jclp.20523

Parth, K., Datz, F., Seidman, C., & Löffler-Stastka, H. (2017). Transference and countertransference: A review. *Bulletin of the Menninger Clinic, 81*(2), 167–211. https://doi.org/10.1521/bumc.2017.81.2.167

Perls, F. S., Goodman, P., & Hefferline, R. F. (1951). *Gestalt therapy: Excitement and growth in the human personality.* Dell.

Pieterse, A. L., Lee, M., Ritmeester, A., & Collins, N. M. (2013). Towards a model of self-awareness development for counselling and psychotherapy training. *Counselling Psychology Quarterly, 26*(2), 190–207. https://doi.org/10.1080/09515070.2013.793451

Rake, C., & Paley, G. (2009). Personal therapy for psychotherapists: The impact on therapeutic practice. A qualitative study using interpretative phenomenological analysis. *Psychodynamic Practice, 15*(3), 275–294. https://doi.org/10.1080/147536 30903024481

Reupert, A. (2006). The counsellor's self in therapy: An inevitable presence. *International Journal for the Advancement of Counselling, 28*(1), 95–105. https://doi. org/10.1007/s10447-005-9001-2

Rizq, R., & Target, M. (2008). 'Not a little Mickey Mouse thing': How experienced counselling psychologists describe the significance of personal therapy in clinical practice and training. Some results from an interpretative phenomenological analysis. *Counselling Psychology Quarterly, 21*(1), 29–48. https://doi.org/10.1080/ 09515070801936578

Rogers, C. R. (1995). What understanding and acceptance mean to me. *Journal of Humanistic Psychology, 35*(4), 7–22. https://doi.org/10.1177/00221678950354002

Shadley, M. L. (2000). Are all therapists alike? Revisiting research about the use of self in therapy. In M. Baldwin (Ed.), *The use of self in therapy* (2nd ed., pp. 191–211). Haworth Press.

Sharma, P., Mehta, M., & Sagar, R. (2017). Efficacy of transdiagnostic cognitive-behavioral group therapy for anxiety disorders and headache in adolescents. *Journal of Anxiety Disorders, 46*, 78–84. https://doi.org/10.1016/j.janxdis.2016.11.001

Siegel, D. J. (2010). *The mindful therapist: A clinician's guide to mindsight and neural integration.* W. W. Norton.

Singhal, M., Munivenkatappa, M., Kommu, J. V., & Philip, M. (2018). Efficacy of an indicated intervention program for Indian adolescents with subclinical depression. *Asian Journal of Psychiatry, 33*, 99–104. https://doi.org/10.1016/j.ajp.2018.03.007

Spagnuolo Lobb, M. (2019). To become a Gestalt psychotherapist within a group: ethics of a teaching/learning community. *New Gestalt Voices, 5*, 31–40.

Staemmler, F. M. (2010). The willingness to be uncertain: Preliminary thoughts about interpretation and understanding in gestalt therapy. In L. Jacobs & R. Hycner (Eds.), *Relational approaches in gestalt therapy* (pp. 65–110). Gestalt Press.

Staemmler, F. M. (2016). Self as a situated process. In J.-M. Robine (Ed.), *Self: Une polyphonie de gestalt-thérapeutes contemporains* (pp. 105–121). L'Exprimerie.

Stawman, S. (2009). Relational gestalt: Four waves. In L. Jacobs & R. Hycner (Eds.), *Relational approaches in gestalt therapy* (pp. 11–36). Gestalt Press.

Tharyan, A. (2000). An experiment in psychotherapy training. *Indian Journal of Psychiatry, 42*(2), 142–147.

Timm, T. M., & Blow, A. J. (1999). Self-of-the-therapist work: A balance between removing restraints and identifying resources. *Contemporary Family Therapy, 21*(3), 331–351. www.wyomingcounselingassociation.com/wp-content/uploads/Timm-Blow-1999-Self-Of-Therapist-Work.pdf.

van Deurzen, E., & Adams, M. (2011). The framework of existential therapy. In *Skills in existential counselling & psychotherapy* (pp. 8–33). SAGE.

Wheeler, G., & Axelsson, L. (2015). *Gestalt therapy.* (J. Carlson & M. Englar-Carlson, Eds.). American Psychological Association.

Yalom, I. D. (1975). *The theory and practice of group psychotherapy* (2nd ed.). Basic Books.

Yalom, I. D. (2002). *The gift of therapy: An open letter to a new generation of therapists and their patients.* HarperCollins.

Yontef, G. (2002). The relational attitude in gestalt therapy theory and practice. *International Gestalt Journal, 25*(1), 15–34.

Yontef, G. (2009). The relational attitude in gestalt therapy and practice. In L. Jacobs & R. Hycner (Eds.), *Relational approaches in gestalt therapy* (pp. 37–59). Gestalt Press.

Yontef, G., & Jacobs, L. (2010). Gestalt Therapy. In R. J. Corsini & D. Wedding (Eds.), *Current psychotherapies* (pp. 342–380). Brooks/Cole.

Yontef, G., & Schulz, F. (2016). Dialogue & experiment. *British Gestalt Journal, 25*(1), 9–21.

Yontef, G. M. (1993). *Awareness, dialogue & process: Essays on gestalt therapy*. Gestalt Journal Press.

Chapter 5

Framework for Facilitating Groups

Holding Environment

Anita was a member of a process-oriented training group that I facilitated many years ago. She was generally on time, and late on rare occasions when she would arrive wounded from minor road accidents on the way. Although skeptical initially, she was earnest in her participation during process work and had a childlike honesty that was endearing. She would often challenge and question the structure of the process-oriented training group—something I found chiefly refreshing, thought provoking and rarely annoying. At times, I would experience her as attacking, sarcastic and confrontational, interspersed with vulnerability, care, honesty and a quest to be seen and cared for by me. After I finished my segment of the course for the training, I did not see her for a while. I met her again a year later when she attended the residential therapy group that I conduct annually. Both she and I struggled with the challenges of wanting to connect, as the attacks and confrontations about my way of running the group continued. This is when the magnitude of her trauma from childhood came to the foreground in her matter-of-fact narrative. I felt pained by her story, where she, the group members and I grieved for her neglected childhood that was replete with experiences of nearly dying. This was followed by a one-year break. I had a sense that the level of vulnerability she felt each time she got close to me and group members needed time to absorb and digest, and I respected the pace at which she wanted to move in her journey.

Anita came back for the retreat again four years ago. She started day one with the old frustration of how she felt stifled by my rules during a feeling check and how rigid I am about closing on time during breaks and at the end of the day. Her experiences in other therapy groups had been very different, and so she found my group format challenging. She said, 'I am not comfortable sitting quietly during a feeling check, I have many thoughts and questions to ask the person sharing and if I don't get to express myself immediately, I lose track [...] why can't you be more flexible about time? I think you want to be in control over things and establish your authority as group leader! You are unwilling to give away power'. This was one, amid many other complaints she had about me.

DOI: 10.4324/9781003348337-6

I quickly became aware of familiar feelings of curiosity, affection, fatigue and annoyance. After listening to her for a while and reflecting on her feelings, I said, 'Yes, I see how this can be stifling for you when I adhere to the rules, especially those related to maintaining the structure of time for sharing and breaks. I do want to find a way out that works for you, the group and me. I feel frustrated when you interrupt, because it takes us away from when someone else is checking in. The idea is to listen, see what comes up for you and share when it's your turn, so everyone in the group gets their equal time to share [...] you are free to share, even when we are breaking for tea, I will leave and be back before break ends'.

During tea break, she and another member, Rema, continued to share their experiences, requesting an additional two minutes. I left and on the way for tea, I demonstrated to some members the concept of 'adjacent possible' on the square tiled floor. Before continuing with the case vignette of Anita, I want to briefly explain the concept of adjacent possible and share my understanding of it through a brief story. Stuart Kauffman (1994), a theoretical biologist, coined the term 'adjacent possible', a theory to explain the biodiversity on earth. He proposes that at any given point, biological systems can only transmute into more intricate systems in certain preset ways. Kauffman's intention was to apply this theory to the origin of life and the development of molecules on Earth. However, the theory has influenced philosophers, psychologists, technologists and social thinkers to understand and describe progress in general. Applying it to psychotherapy, we often observe that awareness, change and growth in life is an incremental process. Each minute step opens up new possibilities. I want to share a childhood experience with you to illustrate the concept further. When I was a little girl, I used to play a game with my older brother, whenever he was sufficiently bored to engage in games with me. This was a fairly common game played by girls across India. In the state I come from, we used to call it kallukali[1] *(a game of stones), where we would draw squares on the ground and hop from box to box pushing a flat stone into the next, with one foot. It required balance, sensory-motor coordination, a high level of concentration and an acute awareness of one's body in relation to one's environment. The rules of the game were that we could only move from one square to the adjacent. Jumping squares and moving either diagonally or straight by skipping adjacent squares was not a possible option. Even if we tried, we would fall flat on our face, given the huge leap one had to make. This is the simplest way I can explain the concept of adjacent possible.*

When the group resumed, Anita and Rema shared how they found my leaving insensitive. I admitted that in an attempt to be sensitive to my need to attend to my bladder or hunger, sometimes I end up being insensitive to others' needs. I was especially sorry about hopping away because in my head it was a break and I was responding to a question from a member about adjacent possibilities and not intending to be disrespectful to Anita and Rema. I processed their experiences, acknowledging that while Anita was able to express her anger with authority figures and group members, Rema shied away from it. I invited other group members to share their experiences and as a group we explored the individual needs for structuring time and managing boundaries. The structure, format and therapeutic frame for the group remained the same, and interestingly, by afternoon that day Anita would be the one to tell us when it was time for a break.

The way I conduct a group is informed by the knowledge I have acquired over the span of my education—mandatory as well as discretionary, personal experiences of being a group member during my training to be a therapist, and my supervised learnings from leading groups. There were many factors that contributed to the ongoing development of Anita's and my awareness, growth and change. I believed that Anita's yearning to heal supported this process of ongoing development, although when I shared this chapter with Anita, she corrected me saying, 'it's not healing I am looking for, I come to the group for understanding and it's the journey that matters to me'. Another important factor that provided a scaffolding was the group's ability to create a safe space that could hold all the upheavals that would be part of many of our group meetings. In addition, my knowledge of guidelines for practicing group therapy from a relational stance helped me hold the frame firmly while being mindful of her hidden vulnerability beneath her expressed anger and pervasive confrontations about my way of conducting the group. An in-depth knowledge about facilitating groups is an indispensable skill for a group leader to be effective under the complex demands of being attentive to the whole group while being attuned to individual members. Feder (1980), discussing the climate of safety and danger in the Gestalt group, says that

> A nurturing, safe-enough group environment is, then, a vital background for meaningful therapeutic work [...] For me as a therapist, any signs or indication that the group as a whole is not a safe place for any or all members result in the climate remerging as a figure, demanding my attention and efforts to establish the necessary levels of safety.
>
> *p. 45*

The vignette 'Holding Environment' emphasizes the importance of following a therapeutic frame for facilitating groups with a phenomenological attitude using Buber's dialogic existentialism. Besides the guidelines for the practice of group therapy, it is crucial to keep in mind the different developmental stages of the group, appropriate interventions, and the role of the group leader to ensure a safe container for the group. Based on the importance of practice guidelines—especially in India, given that we do not have an ethical body governing the practice of group therapy—I have described the ethics in practice, the developmental stages of group and relational interventions, and the role of the group leader. For an in-depth understanding of theory and practice of group therapy, I recommend Yalom's (1995) book, which is a seminal and comprehensive contribution to the informed practice of group therapy, and Levine's (1979) extensive contribution to the practice and development of group psychotherapy. For assimilating Yalom's and Levine's contributions into the practice of GGT, I would recommend books on GGT by Feder and Ronall (1980), Feder and Frew (2008), Feder (2013) and Cole and Reese (2017).

The APA Task Force for Group Psychotherapy (Bernard et al., 2008) have explained two models of practice for group psychotherapy. One model emphasizes empirically supported therapies where treatment interventions are based on the data accrued from randomized clinical trials. These are distinct interventions applied to distinct conditions, like personality disorders. This is a disorder-based approach. A second model of group psychotherapy uses the group setting and relational dynamics as the bedrock for change. This second model is more of a phenomenological approach, which is fluid, flexible and relational in its methodology. In this model the leader is attentive to the three major forces operating in a group—intrapersonal, interpersonal and whole-group dynamic.

The practice guidelines, stages of group development and therapist role and interventions that I have illuminated in this chapter are based on the relational model. To this model I have added my knowledge and experience specific to the practice of GGT in India. The task of the group leader is to be alert to the complex variables that are crucial to the practice and outcome of group therapy. This involves being attentive to ethics, the therapeutic factors, the stages of group development, ego strength of individual members, subjective experiences of individuals as well as the whole group, the group as a whole factor, the sociocultural context of the group members, and the embodied experiences of the leader. The guidelines articulated here are relevant to different group therapy approaches with different kinds of groups, and in a varied treatment setting with amendments based on the participants who have been selected for the group therapy.

Ethics in Group Therapy

Having a set of ethical guidelines and codes of conduct for practicing individual or group therapy is of paramount importance in the field of psychotherapy. Ethics are not enforceable; however, codes of ethics are directives for behavior and require professional adherence. The group leader's knowledge, competencies, skills, values, morals, cultural sensitivity and self-awareness are all crucial factors that regulate ethical practice. Kottler (1994) has emphasized the importance of developing ethical awareness as a group leader because of the complexity, risk of damage and challenges associated with group therapy. Research on the efficacy and outcome of different kinds of therapy groups also highlights the importance of ethical awareness of a group leader (Yalom et al., 1970; Yalom & Lieberman, 1971; Lieberman et al., 1973).

As I mentioned earlier, in India a unified or set standard of ethics in practice with licensure for counseling and psychotherapy or group psychotherapy is yet to be implemented. I think until we can evolve and put into place ethical guidelines for group therapy, it's advisable for us to follow the ethical guidelines set by the psychological associations of other countries and adapt them mindfully to the practice of group therapy within the Indian cultural context. For example, the American Group Psychotherapy Association is an organization that provides ethical guidelines for group therapy to serve professionals in the mental health field (Bernard et al., 2008). Keeping these in mind, I have described below some ethical guidelines for group therapists in India.

Knowledge, Skills and Competencies

Group leaders must be mindful that they have the necessary knowledge, skills, competencies and training to facilitate a group. In addition, I believe that we need to professionally network with our peers and seniors to ensure that we consult with others regarding our work. Preventive measures by leaders must include professional interactions with other therapists, acceptance of the demand for accountability, self-reflection on countertransference and consistent access to supervision (Cole & Reese, 2017; Leszcz, 2004; Yalom, 1995).

While allowing the group to unfold and minimizing one's control over the way the group evolves, leaders must be able to intervene when there is abuse of one member by the other, and identify high-risk members and members who can cause damage. Members in therapy groups can unknowingly engage in scapegoating, damaging and shaming confrontation, and inappropriate reassurance (Corey & Corey, 1997). I think this includes the leader, too. As group leaders we should be aware of how we relate with each member as well be able to intervene to minimize unhelpful behaviors that can lead to shame, isolation, fear and inauthentic ways of being that are counterproductive in the long run. I think our consultations, as well as engaging in dialogue with the members about the genesis and real emotions behind these behaviors is an important relational intervention. In addition, by practicing inclusion, we increase the chances of role modeling helpful interpersonal skills. I usually intervene by asking the member who is attacking or reassuring, what they are feeling in this group, exploring what they hope and fear. For example, in a group I facilitated, a male participant named Rakesh took an instant dislike to a female participant, Remya, whom he experienced as an aggressive feminist activist. Remya was hurt and puzzled by Rakesh's hostility toward her. Some of the other female participants tried hard to please him, offering validation and reassurances. When I explored what was happening with each of the group members, what emerged was Rakesh's fear of women, whom he experienced as aggressive, triggering memories of his mother whom he was scared of. Remya's experiences were of having been victimized as a girl while growing up and her rage toward patriarchy. The female participants who tried to reassure Rakesh had developed an antenna for how to please male figures in the hope of being accepted for being docile, yet they felt anger toward male figures that they were afraid of expressing. These explorations were ongoing, and over time members developed an awareness of how their past experiences colored their perceptions of their present ways of relating with each other. My personal reflections about how our life experiences and culture shape us, and consultations with my supervisor gave me the support to process these interpersonal issues.

In the absence of sufficient competency and supervision, I believe leaders can unknowingly miss some of these group dynamics, which can impair the building of awareness and find resolution for interpersonal conflicts. Lack of skill and competency can also lead to leader behaviors that can be highly problematic, and may include being coercive with members to disclose, or failing to acknowledge when one has been party to causing damage to members. As group leaders, we should be conscious of the potential for misusing power in the group, especially so in our cultural context, which is steeped in caste, class, religion and gender hierarchy. Moreover, a disturbing issue we face in India is undergraduate students, beginner practitioners, diploma holders and alternative healing practitioners conducting therapy/growth groups—mostly unsupervised, and with limited/no knowledge and skills in conducting groups.

Screening and Selection

The screening process for the selection of the therapy group is very important. If it's not done effectively, there is a risk of bringing members into the group who may not be in a psychological space to be part of the group. There are instances when I have faced this challenge, especially while conducting growth groups for counseling institutes and government organizations. In one such instance, halfway into the group therapy, I realized the vulnerability of one of the participants named Radha, while another participant, Amita, was relating her experiences of domestic violence and abuse. It led to Radha suffering a breakdown and showing symptoms of severe trauma. Although I spent time holding and containing the stress responses, I could barely manage to emotionally soothe Radha in the group space. This left a disturbing impact on the other group members. Even though Radha showed signs of quick recovery, I suspect some damage was done to her by being part of this therapy group.

Individuals usually benefit from individual therapy; however, it is fairly deducible that not all individuals benefit from group therapy. In fact, therapeutic groups can directly contribute to adverse outcomes for some clients, including the experience of enduring psychological distress attributable to one's group experience (Yalom & Leszcz, 2005). I believe my failure to engage in a thorough screening, and complacency about Radha being part of a counselor training institute contributed to this mishap and I still carry regret over this.

Confidentiality

Confidentiality is easier to be assured of in an individual setting, whereas in group therapy this has limitations. Therapists should discuss with potential group members the problem of protecting clients' confidentiality from one another, since confidentiality in group settings is not something a leader can guarantee. Although I encourage group members to maintain confidentiality and not share experiences of other group members with anybody outside the group, I also talk about the challenges of enforcing this in a group. I find it helpful to encourage group members to own the responsibility for confidentiality. I can't recollect any problems related to confidentiality in the groups I have conducted so far. However, if you remember the story 'Survivors' narrated in chapter 3, in which I was a group participant, the lack of communication by the leader about confidentiality and the absence of informed consent for using what emerged in the group for research purposes did impact the way the members felt about safety. This personal experience has helped me be mindful about issues around confidentiality, educate group members and make the conversations around it an ongoing process in the group.

Structure and Boundaries

Consistently maintaining the boundaries related to time, fees, ways of communicating and relating with each other are all crucial, as related in the vignette 'Holding Environment'. Leaders need to be committed to understanding the meanings of individual and group actions that disturb the therapeutic frame. However, rigidly refusing to cross a boundary that may be appropriate and therapeutic in a specific context could also have a detrimental effect on the therapeutic relationship (Barnett, 1998). I remember one instance with Anita in which she was curious to understand how I was feeling after my father's death, which occurred around the time of one of our residential retreats, and I shared with her some of my feelings of grief. When I checked with her how my sharing landed on her, she came back with the response that 'somehow it made you human and I saw your vulnerable side, it made me feel more connected to you and OK with my vulnerabilities…'

Dual Relationships

We all know by now that dual relationships can be complex and problematic, and we also know that within the Indian cultural context dual relationships are often unavoidable, given that the numbers of trained professionals available for teaching, supervision and therapy are dismally limited compared to the demands of the growing field. During my own training to be a therapist, more than two decades ago, my trainers were also my supervisors and therapists. The situation is much better now in some training institutes with demarcations around dual roles. However, we are still learning through trial and error with our scarce resources.

Duality may arise in group therapy in circumstances when therapists and members have academic or supervisory relationships with each other, when group members or leaders have outside contact with each other in a social context, and when multiple roles exist between the group leader and the group member. In my training groups that are process oriented, many of my trainees have attended the residential retreat I conduct specifically for practitioners. Although it's not mandatory to attend nor does their evaluation depend on it, it can still pose some challenges for us. I have tried to minimize these challenges by ensuring that their supervision for their practice is done by other professionals in the field and the evaluations are based only on their supervised practice, formal assessment and peer feedback. The American Psychological Association's (APA's) ethical code emphasizes that students participating in group therapy as a part of training should not be evaluated by academic faculty related to such therapy (cite Standard 7.05, APA, 2002).

Record Keeping and Consulting

Record keeping should be adhered to while protecting individual members' confidentiality. The records also help during regular consultations with one's supervisor to maintain professionalism, rationale for interventions and to also explore one's own unavoidable countertransference feelings. This kind of rigor helps in maintaining ethics in practice while facilitating groups, and in the long run it strengthens the practitioner's awareness, skills and competencies. Although this may not be directly correlated to group therapy outcome, I believe that it supports and enhances the quality of work that the leader brings into the therapy setting.

I have briefly explained some critical ethical guidelines above, based on my knowledge and experiences as a group therapist. I strongly recommend additional readings and adherence to the guidelines that support best global practices in group therapy (Bernard et al., 2008; Levine, 1979; Yalom et al., 1970; Yalom & Lieberman, 1997; Yalom & Leszcz, 2005)

Role of the Group Leader

I think by now it's fairly clear the importance of the 'self' of the therapist, both in individual and group therapy, given the extent of the literature available about the importance of therapist qualities. As therapists we need to be fairly clear that creative growth and change in the other are influenced by the leader's attunement, sensitivity in action and ability to engage using their creative potential. Many practitioners have emphasized the group leader's role and ability to be present and the impact of lack of ability and awareness. One valuable contribution to understanding the role of a group leader is that of Lieberman et al. (1973). Although more than 40 years have passed since their research findings, it is equally relevant today. Lieberman and his colleagues set up 18 encounter, process, growth and training groups, studied their experiences and compared the outcome. The groups represented some major theoretical approaches, including those of the basic National Training Laboratory, GT, Transactional Analysis, Esalen eclectic, personal growth, Synanon, psychodrama, marathon, encounter groups, and a psychoanalytically oriented group, at the end of which participant experiences were elicited.

The findings from the study suggests that the ideal leader of a group is moderate in their amount of emotional stimulation, shows executive behavior in caring for the members of their group, and uses certain cognitive functions to help make meaning of the group's experiences. They identified four basic roles of the leader: Executive function, Caring, Emotional stimulation and Meaning-attribution. The authors have pointed out the importance of the leader's assessment skills, being aware and committed to their responsibilities, caring for the group, role modeling effective behavior, and an ability to balance feelings with thinking functions in dealing with the group.

The leader must possess a considerable amount of knowledge concerning the group process and the leader's role. The damaging leadership style was categorized by high stimulus input, aggressivity, charisma, support, intrusiveness and individual rather than group focus. Leaders who demand more feelings through provocative, challenging and stimulating behavior were, on average, likely to induce more casualties. Although the leadership functions may vary from group to group, depending on the setting in which the leader works, these factors given by them are crucial parameters to consider in group practice.

It's important to be cognizant of the stages of group development proposed by different theoreticians, and the therapeutic factors proposed by Yalom (1995) that improve the outcome of group therapy. While working with each group, I focus more on the phenomenology of each member, the sociocultural context I work in and my own embodied experiences. This helps me to be open to what emerges in the here and now, and be curious about the unexpected rather than expecting what has been theorized. I agree with Fairfield (2004) that generally group therapists have used Yalom's (1995) model as an instructional manual, which can lead to the therapist missing what is contrary to this. The risk of this increases especially when applied to cultures that are different, where this model needs to be adapted to suit the context. Hence, it's important to have an in-depth understanding of GT and apply it in group practice as its basic philosophical premise supports mindfulness to diversity.

Beginning the Circle: Guidelines for Structuring a Group

My work begins when I am invited to facilitate a group—these groups can be for members within the psychotherapy community like counseling students and trainees; for institutions that conduct growth groups for teachers, priests and nuns; and for trauma-focused therapy, like groups for trafficked girls. I spend a fair amount of time understanding the stakeholders and their expectations so that I can have a tentative framework for facilitating the group. Usually, the objective of the stakeholders is to build self-awareness, cope with trauma and reduce interpersonal conflicts.

Engaging Multiple Stakeholders

Depending on the requirements of the stakeholders, the frequency, hours and duration of the sessions are decided. Collaborative relationships with government officers, institute administrators and managers are important. They are vital stakeholders because they are the ones who have requested group therapy for their staff/members of the organization, and our relationship with them has an impact on the work we do with the primary clients. Creating therapy groups that have the potential to be successful involves active engagement between the clients, therapist and administrators.

I remember while working with trafficked girls, it was fairly common for a few of the girls to run away from the institution with an adult perpetrator. The official in charge would feel quite angry and disappointed when this occurred. On one such occasion, I decided to sit with them sharing tea, listening to their disappointments. Then I responded with,

> you have spent most of your life dedicated to rescuing and providing a safe home for these children. It must be painful to see some of them going back to a life that is scary for you. This work is really challenging for us; we are often grieving for the children we lose.

They cried and spoke about their own childhood where there was not much protection and how they yearned for it and how it hurt them that the girls run away for sex. Toward the end of that informal conversation, I shared with them my sense that often it's not about sex, that there are many complex factors that are at play here, and that 'it's the only touch they are familiar with while growing up, and when there is a loss of that for such a prolonged period, they may in desperation go back to the perpetrator'. I am not sure if this drastically changed the way they viewed the girls who ran away; however, they were supportive of the work I did with the children and would personally look forward to my visits and our shared ritual of tea.

Our work as group therapists needs to expand to the larger field and context, especially if we want to see our work with specific groups bring about change in the wider social web to which we belong as human beings. If we can hold the system that comprises the stakeholders with compassion, then there is a possibility of improving the support resources for our clients. Moreover, we must be mindful about the possibility that the stakeholders were children once upon a time with their share of trauma and capacity for childlike hope.

Preparing Group Members for the Therapeutic Frame

The group leader must be clear and transparent to the group members about the structure and framework of the group. I usually communicate through writing the important rules and norms before the commencement of the program, as well as directly on the first day of the group meeting. For example, this would include communications related to fees, time, duration, consent, confidentiality, venue, the size of the group, the background of the group facilitator and co-facilitator (if present), participation in the group and absences or leaving the group prematurely. Yalom and Leszcz (2005) recommend that before the group commences, key aspects of appropriate group participation, including self-disclosure, interpersonal feedback, confidentiality, extra-group contact and the parameters of termination need to be defined and communicated. This is reiterated by GGT practitioners too (Cole & Reese, 2017; Feder & Ronall, 1980; Feder & Frew, 2008). The better informed that individuals are about the objectives and processes of the group, the easier will be their understanding, engagement, work, attendance and commitment to the group process.

Communication of Goals

I don't have any specific goals that I form before starting a group. I am attentive to what the stakeholders want; however, I also encourage the group members to formulate what they are looking for from being in the group. Because most of the groups I have facilitated so far already have preset goals around building self-awareness, interpersonal skills and developing skills of empathy, it's easier for me to go in with a tentative set of objectives and then let the group members and I together create the intersubjective field from which their goals get further clarified.

I start the first meeting of the group usually with a feeling check, discussing expectations and exploring fears. Here I use the 'talking stick' as a metaphor for providing opportunity to each member to share their feelings without interruptions or intellectual questioning. After the sharing and self-reflective listening, the members are free to come back to how each person's sharing impacted them personally and to build a tentative contract for what they would want to work on. This helps me get to know the group members better and also set a ground rule about the importance of being silently reflective. I also share how I am feeling, because it's important for me to flow between my role as a group leader as well as be what Yalom (1995) calls a 'fellow-traveler'. In addition, I have found from personal experience, some level of self-disclosure helps in modeling openness, minimizing hierarchy and encouraging self-reflection.

Stages of Group Development

Many theoreticians and practitioners of group therapy have hypothesized about the different stages that groups go through (Bernard et al., 2008; Feder &Frew, 2008; Garland et al., 1973; Kepner, 1980; Levine, 1979; Spagnuolo Lobb, 2013; Yalom, 1995) and they all share certain commonalities. (Schutz, 1966 cited in Kepner, 1980) suggested that there were three categories of needs people bring into groups, and these needs, while interrelated, tend to emerge in a hierarchical order or in stages—the need to affiliate or to belong, the need for autonomy and the need for affection. On an emotional level, these needs are experienced as issues around identity, power and intimacy. The need to belong and to establish one's identity produces dependent behavior; the need for autonomy makes the individual test out the limits of authority, and produces counterdependent behavior; and the need for intimacy motivates people to relate interdependently. Zinker (Feder & Ronall, 1980), distinguishes four stages of what he calls the group cycle: exploration, identity, isolation, high cohesion. Hodges (2003) gives a five-stage model of Orientation, Power and control, Intimacy, Differentiation and Termination to map out how the group configures, with each stage having different needs that emerge in the group and tasks for the leader.

Kepner (1980) identified three stages of group development—each stage marked by certain developmental tasks that are crucial for growth and change. They are Identity and Dependence, Influence and Counterdependence, Intimacy and Interdependence. She elaborates on these stages by giving examples of the hopes and fears that the members feel in groups, suggesting tasks for the leaders to support these. She says that GT when practiced relationally, differs noticeably from the traditional GT as practiced by Perls and some of his followers, which was individual therapy done in a group setting. Perls suggested that there were three categories of needs people bring into groups, and these needs, while interrelated, tend to emerge in a hierarchical order: the need to affiliate or to belong; the need for autonomy; and the need for affection. On an emotional level, these needs are experienced as issues around identity, power and intimacy. The need to belong and to establish one's identity produces dependent behavior; the need for autonomy makes the individual test out the limits of authority and produces counterdependent behavior; and the need for intimacy motivates people to relate interdependently. Kepner connects Erikson's psychosocial stages for individual development to the stages of group development and says that the same principles can be applied to group development. This implies that the developmental tasks of the previous stage need to be met adequately for the tasks of the next stage to be addressed or dealt with. For example, the need for belongingness needs to be met adequately before a member can safely move into self-disclosure.

Another theory that greatly appeals to me and that I keep in mind while working with groups is transactional analyst Levin-Landheer's (1982) developmental stages, where she proposes the cycles of development that recur throughout the life span of a human being. She postulates that human growth goes through cycles of development, which begin in infancy and repeat throughout life like a spiral. She talks about the stages that a human being goes through from birth that includes being, doing, thinking, identity formation, being skillful, regeneration and recycling. Using Erikson's developmental stages as a foundation, she proposes that the infant goes through developmental cycles with needs for trust, autonomy and identity as they move toward adolescence. Around the age of 12, the adolescent recycles all these needs and has the opening to meet the unmet yearnings of infancy and childhood. I believe that these essential needs, emotional yearnings for attunement appear over and over, again and again, and one has opportunities in the environment for being met in relation with another. I think, in a therapeutic setting awareness of the cyclic nature of unmet developmental needs gives an opening for both client and therapist to be attuned and find ways to meet the needs to an approximation.

Her theory really appeals to me. It resonates with my way of working because it offers flexibility in viewing the group stages as fluid with growth as well as with setbacks. Thus, it keeps us open to whatever is emerging moment to moment that fits into the phenomenological field approach of GT. The group goes through cycles in its developmental needs for being, doing, thinking, identity formation and recycling. Often members may be at different stages of developmental needs and an understanding of each member's yearnings and the group as a whole can help the leader provide appropriate interventions. It is important to keep in mind that these stages follow a cycle of development and the demarcations are not necessarily distinct and rigid; rather, they are fluid, flexible and interconnected.

Combining the individual and group development theories proposed by different theoreticians, we can gain insight into the stages of group development enabling informed interventions. This model implies that the leader's role and interventions need to change based on the developmental stages of the group over time. The stages I have described below are based on different models of stages of group development and my personal experiences of working with groups.

Nascent Anxiety and Dependence

Individuals come in for therapy with some level of anxiety related to how the therapist will be, a sense of inadequacy for not fixing their problems, and often shame about having problems in the first place. These anxieties are accompanied by concerns about inclusion and exclusion in the group, fears around belongingness and concerns around one's safety. 'Being' is vulnerable and anxious, 'doing' is accompanied with a dread of being judged and a hope of being accepted, and 'thinking' is mostly internal—marked by reticence about whether it is safe to express in the group. The identity of each member of the group relies, to some degree, on the way in which they are perceived and responded to by every other member of the group, including the leader.

Frew (1997) suggests that the individual member in a group organizes their perceptions of the field moment to moment, and a particular aspect of the field becomes figural for the member at a given time. For example, Frew (1997) says that at the beginning of the group, a member may want to know, 'How much time and resources do I need to invest in this group, how long will this last, how will this help me to cope better in my life?' If the group leader provides a structure, framework, principles and guidelines in a clear transparent manner, then this concern that was 'figural' recedes into the ground and something else comes up in awareness to be attended to. This could be the need for 'being': 'How safe am I in this group? Will I be understood? Can I trust the leader to really care for me?' (p. 134). If the leader intervenes through a felt sense, explores and affirms these concerns with openness, and demonstrates genuine warmth and care, then there is a possibility of trust development. This figure formation process, completion of a Gestalt and emergence of a new Gestalt is an ongoing process that group leaders can be attentive to during the different stages of GGT.

Gestalt therapists see this figure formation as closely linked to the Gestalt concept of organismic self-regulation, whether it be with individual or group therapy. The organism or the individual is in relation to the field and will try to regulate or meet their needs in the best way possible under the given conditions. Within the group, each individual, including the leader, is attempting to regulate their needs based on what is figural for that individual. This may not be a conscious part for each group member, but it is important that the leader is conscious about the leader's own needs, roles, responsibilities, emotional space, bodily sensations and sense of what group members may be experiencing.

Interventions. This is the stage where the group leader needs to clarify the purpose of the group; set a contract for timing, duration, fees, and communications related to being present in the group; and demarcate boundaries and provide information about the way the leader is going to approach the tasks at hand. The leader also facilitates the development of relationships with the members while creating a safe and warm containing space. Usually in this stage, the members are more dependent on the leader and may prefer to interact more with the leader. I, typically, begin a group by communicating clearly my stance on relationality, the way I work with groups, the rules, norms and guidelines. I am attentive to each member's name and what they have checked in as their feelings and expectations. I structure some expressive art activity through which the members can express their experiences individually. This is followed by large group sharing. The activities are geared toward self-reflection, and taking small steps toward interpersonal trust. Since self-disclosure is likely to be scary in the early stages, I leave it to each member how much of their experiences they want to share in the larger group.

I try to be attuned to how the group is forming—whether members spend excessive time philosophizing, or continue to stay disconnected from each other. I reflect on how I experience this phenomenon and wonder what role I play in maintaining this. What I do as a response is to experiment with a different way of being, action or an opposing idea or philosophy. For example, I may suggest that each person share what they feel about connection and disconnection, or feeling 'whole' or fragmented in their bodies. Then I process what comes up. Usually, idealizing the leader is high at this stage, I have learned over time and through my supervisions to manage the feelings of unease this creates in me and neither challenge it nor allow this to feed my narcissistic needs.

Acute Anxiety and Counterdependence

At this stage, members become more aware of how each impacts the other, and may feel comfort or threat in the norms and rules that place a restriction on individual freedom. There is an implicit requirement to regulate one's behavior to accommodate what is valued, permissible or acceptable in a group. Some members may challenge the rules by expressing discontent or by interrupting. The leader can be experienced as a parental figure, whose authority and control are intimidating. Some members may struggle to express these feelings directly. I believe that this could stem from the cultural factors that dissuade individuals from showing disagreement with authority figures given the hierarchical structure. I also see this as the individual's creative ways of expressing a need and the anxiety attached to it. Directly questioning the authority of the leader, in my experience, in an Indian group setting is very rare. The challenges are usually more passive—showing compliance and shying away from questioning because challenging the hierarchy is accompanied with fear or/and guilt.

This stage is marked by increased anxiety associated often with an intensified need to belong, and an equally palpable dread of injury from attachments. As the group meetings progress, competitiveness, rivalry akin to those between siblings, and hostile conflicts with members may become figural. Formation of subgroups and out-groups are quite common, especially in the

Indian context. We need to be deeply attuned to these cultural dynamics and find ways to intervene that minimize shame triggers. Anita is an exception to the groups I have conducted, and even for her the confrontations would be usually followed by anxiety about being rejected. This is something she has shared whenever I have asked her how she feels about challenging me. I have also observed that in the group Anita is part of, other members have been able to express their disappointments with me openly. I have felt appreciative of the energy and creativity that Anita brings into the group. She sets the tone for other members and groups in general to explore their anger/aggression that is held in check.

Interventions. As leaders, we need to be attentive to how anxiety is expressed and dealt with by individual members in the group, and how the lack of expression impacts safety and cohesiveness. As themes around agreements and disagreements about norms, rules and relational dynamics of the group become figural, the leader must encourage expression of the differences that occur at the individual, interpersonal and group level. Facilitating expressions of counterdependence is regulated by the extent of the leader's awareness, cultural experiences, beliefs and attitude toward hierarchy. As group leaders, if we believe that we must be treated with deference because of our role, then it can be problematic for relational work in the Indian group therapy setting. How differences and emotional expressions get dealt with also depends on the ego strength of the individual members and the group as a whole.

The ability to identify roles that members play is another important factor to keep in mind as a leader. Often in groups, just as in family systems, members get entrenched in patterns of behavior like the caretaker, nurturer, scapegoat, victim, persecutor, rescuer, lost child, entertainer, creative impulsive challenger, and the volunteer who does more personal work. These are important functions; however, when it gets set in rigid roles, it can stunt the growth of individual members as well as the group. The leader can bring this to the awareness of the group by making it more figural.

For example, in many of the groups I have conducted where male members are present, they are often treated with extra nurturance or hostility by some female members. When I explore this dynamic further, the group as a whole develops awareness into how culture has shaped beliefs around gratifying the boys' needs more, and internalized patriarchy and anger toward men. When I ask the women members, 'How do you feel nurtured? Who nurtures you? What's your experience of being nurtured in this moment', it is often responded to with an emerging yearning to be nurtured and cared for, and there is grief and anger about having missed it in their early experiences as well as in the present context.

The leader also needs to be attuned to how each person operates from their shadow self, and for this process to work well, the leader needs to be in touch with their own shadow parts that lie outside conscious awareness (Cole & Reese, 2017). The shadow self as a concept was first coined by Carl Jung to describe aspects of our personality that we are not aware of, or reject in ourselves. For example, a tendency to be aggressive with people who are in a subordinate position of power can be our way of coping with our feelings of helplessness or of being devalued. Often what troubles us painfully in others is the parts of ourselves that we have disowned and feel ashamed about. For example, in a therapy group that I conducted, gratitude as a theme came up for Fae, and how disappointed she feels when she experiences others as ungrateful. In this situation, I started my invitation for an experiment embedded in a dialogue:

VANAJA: I get that gratitude is a very important value for you, and I have experienced you expressing your gratitude on many occasions within this group and to me.

FAE: (Nods her head, then looks at me thoughtfully, head tilted slightly to her shoulder). Yes, it's an important value for me.

VANAJA: I resonate with your value and I can see how disturbed you feel when you experience others not sharing this value.

FAE: (smiles hesitantly). I feel disappointed and a judgment comes up.

VANAJA: I personally feel shame when I think I am being ungrateful. How do you feel about what I just shared with you?

FAE: Yes, thank you for sharing [...] I feel a loosening of the judgment [...]

VANAJA: I have an idea; would you like to give it a shot?

I asked Fae if she would want to express the things that she feels grateful and ungrateful about. After the exercise, when I processed her experience, she said that she had never thought about the parts of her that feel ungrateful, and she wasn't aware she had that side. Fae felt vulnerable about showing this side. However, what helped her was her bond with group members, with me and my own self-disclosure. In addition, when I used the word 'value' and shared my observations of her demonstration of this value of gratitude by her on various occasions, she felt comforted that being ungrateful doesn't nullify the essence of her being grateful. This opened the group members toward expressing things they feel grateful and ungrateful about, and the individual shame about one's disowned parts was held and shared by the group.

The leader's interventions at this stage must be geared toward exploring the emotions, identifying unresolved issues in family dynamics that surface in the group, and examining the individual, cultural and universal polarities of being human. As in the vignette about Fae, there were familial expectations about gratitude and Buddhist practices that contributed to her unique ways of being in this world. On the one hand, her values gave Fae a way of relating with others gently, but on the other hand, it curtailed her from tolerating lack of gratitude in herself, which came out as judgments toward people whom she experienced as ungrateful. This was further compounded by shame about being judgmental. While facilitating awareness and contact with the self, we must balance it with interpersonal learning in the group, and confront compassionately when necessary.

Intimacy and Interdependence

This is the stage when the leader is perceived as more human, a less idealized figure, and more as an experienced support to be accessed when needed. Our role as a leader is less active and we may need to step in only when there is a requirement to regulate interpersonal interactions or feedback, continue to build awareness, and facilitate members ability to creatively adjust to patterned ways of responding to problems. If we have facilitated individual awareness and interpersonal conflict management, the members relate with each other proactively for the functioning of the group as a system. The leadership function gets shared by the members of the group. They are active in 'doing'—experimenting with novel ways of problem-solving and enjoying their autonomy to act without the leader's support.

There is role flexibility among members and the leader, and the group is open to less hierarchical and more equitable relationships. Real intimacy and contact are apparent in the group interactions, and the ability to nurture self and sustain relationships gets forged. I have noticed a marked ability in individual members to be vulnerable, engage in self-disclosure, share differing opinions and express honestly to each other without getting triggered into toxic shame. In fact, the awareness to recognize shame and talk about it without feeling shame about one's own shame is often present. At this stage, members are interdependent and they are less likely to shame themselves for their need for dependence and independence. They are able to regulate their needs in the given moment, and empathic attunement to the self and the other has been strengthened.

Interventions. Here the leader's interventions are minimal in terms of letting the group work with each other and continue to develop their awareness. I may intervene if required, to facilitate acceptance of individual differences and realize the capacity to still sustain relationships despite these differences. I step in when I sense the need to introduce an experiment for any group member or the group as a whole that I believe will support individual or group needs. However, I often allow the group to unfold and sustain each other. I have observed that if the group has reached this space, then I actually tend to bodily step back—curl up in my chair more often, remain silent and stay in the fringes as a supportive presence. This happens usually with the groups that I have conducted for three or more years. I have not observed this stage of interdependence in the groups I have conducted for brief durations.

Separation and Termination

During this stage, the members are likely to move toward what the ending of the group means to each one of them. This is the time that the loss and grief related specifically to this ending comes up. In the larger context, past endings as well as the existential reality of loss and grief is also likely to arise. It is important for the leader to prompt from and process with the members the grief of termination as well as the gifts gained from the group. It is unlikely that the individual needs or group needs have all been met at the end of the group. In fact, in many short-term groups, the stage of interdependency, cohesiveness and intimacy has not been fully established. However, if we look at this from the Gestalt perspective the best possible ending has been reached for this group, given the duration of the therapy group, individual member and group awareness and the human limitations of the leader. This completion of a Gestalt has opened up the possibility of another Gestalt, either in the form of individual therapy or the beginning of a new group. I have occasionally had some members tell me that they felt dissatisfied with their expectations not being met, and they did not get full closure for the struggles they experienced. This is especially common during four-day residentials. I accept that as a given of the limitation of this kind of work. When they have returned for the next residential, I have found that their experience has changed, and they have developed an awareness of the incremental nature of healing and change.

Sometimes, self-protective mechanisms can come up for some members who are pained by the termination process because it can trigger old anxieties around loss, grief and maybe even death. This could be a sign that for this particular member the separation is too premature. The leader needs to ensure that these members have access to individual therapy or other forms of support.

Interventions. The leader's primary task is to assist with the expression of feelings around termination and loss. The leader can help members focus on the current ending in the here and now, and may even explore past experiences of termination based on the available time. I usually talk about the upcoming termination a few sessions in advance so that there is opportunity for members to reflect and share their feelings over the next few sessions. This can also help consolidate at a slow pace the similarities and differences in how the members respond to endings. In addition, the leader can encourage reflections on what they have received, what they have given and what needs were unmet in this group. This provides an opportunity to bolster what has been assimilated and also acknowledge and be attentive to unfinished business. I invite members to share the expectations they came in with and where they are at the end. I share what working with this group has meant to me, what I have learned and my joy of having been with them, as well as the sadness of termination.

Gift giving, the sharing of food and celebrations are often helpful to bond, bid goodbye and share gratitude, especially in the Indian cultural context that celebrates numerous festivals and different cuisines across religions and regions. This helps facilitate a warm and celebratory farewell—a reparative experience for past goodbyes that may have been distressing. This is also evocative of archetypal experiences of birth, death and renewal of life.

Group therapy also provides members with the opportunity of mourning the loss of many relationships while still in the company of others who share this lived experience. It may also provide an opening to ask profound existential questions about life—the meaning one makes of togetherness and isolation. The gains from this specific togetherness as part of a group bring the realization that isolation is an inevitable part of being human. It opens up unique meanings for sustaining connections with the self and the other.

I have described the above stages and interventions that the leader can be mindful of based on my experiences with conducting different kinds of groups and what group therapists and theoreticians have said about the stages of group development. However, as a note of caution, this framework must be lightly held as a map, and flexibly changed with each group and at each stage. I have experienced in my work times when the stages don't follow what has been normatively prescribed, and what appeared cohesive has collapsed into chaos, and trust and intimacy has moved into anxiety, isolation and mistrust. The lesson I have learned is to be prepared with the compass of knowledge and competency and be open to navigating with the stars. To quote Kepner (1980), 'What I have done in this paper is to sketch out a map of the territory. Anyone who has travelled knows that a map is not the territory: It is a two-dimensional abstraction of a three-dimensional reality' (p. 10).

Note

1 Kallukali: hopscotch

References

American Psychological Association. (2002). Ethical principles of psychologists and code of conduct. *American Psychologist, 57*(12), 1060–1073. https://doi.org/10.1037/0003-066x.57.12.1060

Barnett, J. E. (1998). Should psychotherapists self-disclose? Clinical and ethical considerations. In L. Vandecreek, S. Knapp, & T. L. Jackson (Eds.), *Innovations in clinical practice: A source book* (pp. 419–428). Professional Resource Exchange.

Bernard, H., Burlingame, G., Flores, P., Greene, L., Joyce, A., Kobos, J. C., Leszcz, M., MacNair-Semands, R. R., Piper, W. E., McEneaney, A. M., & Feirman, D. (2008). Clinical practice guidelines for group psychotherapy. *International Journal of Group Psychotherapy, 58*(4), 455–542. https://doi.org/10.1521/ijgp.2008.58.4.455

Cole, P. H., & Reese, D. A. (2017). *New directions in gestalt group therapy: Relational ground, authentic self.* Routledge.

Corey, M. S., & Corey, G. (1997). *Groups: Process and practice* (5th ed.). Brooks/Cole.

Fairfield, M. A. (2004). Gestalt groups revisited: A phenomenological approach. *Gestalt Review, 8*(3), 336–357. https://doi.org/10.5325/gestaltreview.8.3.0336

Feder, B. (1980). Safety and danger in the gestalt group. In B. Feder & R. Ronall (Eds.), *Beyond the hot seat: Gestalt approaches to group* (pp. 41–52). Brunner/Mazel.

Feder, B. (2013). *Gestalt group therapy: A practical guide* (2nd ed.). CreateSpace Independent Publishing Platform.

Feder, B., & Frew, J. (Eds.). (2008). *Beyond the hot seat revisited: Gestalt approaches to group.* Gestalt Institute of New Orleans.

Feder, B., & Ronall, R. (Eds.). (1980). *Beyond the hot seat: Gestalt approaches to group.* Brunner/Mazel.

Frew, J. E. (1997). A gestalt therapy theory application to the practice of group leadership. *Gestalt Review, 1*(2), 131–149. www.jstor.org/stable/44394034.

Garland, J., Jones, H., & Kolodny, R. (1973). A model for stages of development in social work groups. In S. Bernstein (Ed.), *Explorations in group work: Essays in theory and practice* (pp. 17–71). Milford House.

Hodges, C. (2003). Creative processes in gestalt group therapy. In M. Spagnuolo Lobb & N. Amendt-Lyon (Eds.), *Creative license: The art of gestalt therapy* (pp. 249–259). Springer.

Kauffman, S. A. (1994). *The origins of order: Self-organization and selection in evolution.* Oxford University Press.

Kepner, E. (1980). Gestalt group process. In B. Feder & R. Ronall (Eds.), *Beyond the hot seat: Gestalt approaches to group* (pp. 5–24). Brunner/Mazel.

Kottler, J. A. (1994). Working with difficult group members. *Journal for Specialists in Group Work, 19*(1), 3–10. https://doi.org/10.1080/01933929408413757

Leszcz, M. (2004). Reflections on the abuse of power, control and status in group therapy and group therapy training. *International Journal of Group Psychotherapy, 54*(3), 389–400. https://doi.org/10.1521/ijgp.54.3.389.40343

Levin-Landheer, P. (1982). The cycle of development. *Transactional Analysis Journal, 12*(2), 129–139. https://doi.org/10.1177/036215378201200207

Levine, B. (1979). *Group psychotherapy: Practice and development.* Prentice-Hall.

Lieberman, M. A., Miles, M. B., & Yalom, I. D. (1973). *Encounter groups: First facts.* Basic Books.

Schutz, W. (1966). *The interpersonal underworld.* Science and Behavior Books.

Spagnuolo Lobb, M. (2013). *The now-for-next in psychotherapy: Gestalt therapy recounted in post-modern society.* Istituto Di Gestalt HCC Italy. www.gestaltitaly.com.

Yalom, I. D. (1971). A study of encounter group casualties. *Archives of General Psychiatry, 25*(1), 16–30. https://doi.org/10.1001/archpsyc.1971.01750130018002

Yalom, I. D. (1995). *The theory and practice of group psychotherapy* (4th ed.). Basic Books.

Yalom, I. D., Fidle, J. W., Frank, J., Mann, J., & Sata, L. (1970). Encounter groups and psychiatry: American Psychiatric Association task force report. *American Psychiatric Association, 21*(9). https://doi.org/10.1176/ps.21.9.308-b

Yalom, I. D., & Leszcz, M. (2005). *The theory and practice of group psychotherapy* (5th ed.). Basic Books.

Zinker, J. C. (1980). The developmental process of a gestalt therapy group. In B. Feder & R. Ronall (Eds.), *Beyond the hot seat: Gestalt approaches to group* (pp. 55–77). Brunner/Mazel.

Chapter 6

Phenomenology, Field Theory and Adjacent Possible

Colliding Subjectivities

I pick up the vignette of Anita, where I left it in the last chapter, to trace the development of awareness and change that emerged over the years in the therapy group that she was part of. I spoke about the recurrent struggle we faced regarding the therapeutic frame that I follow while conducting the group. In the residential retreat that Anita attended around four years ago, she had shared that she felt stifled by my rules. Her discomfort with structure and time had come up in past group meetings; however, this was the first time she gave expression to the extent of the frustration she felt with me. Although I invited her to talk more about this experience, she took time and during the second half of the day, she opened up to respond to my questions. What emerged was her memories as a toddler, of being left alone to play with some toys, in a bucket half-filled with water. She recalled experiences of slipping and falling into the bucket, getting bruised and picking herself back up. When asked about how she felt sharing this now, she responded that it was fun for her to play in the water initially; however, she would call out for someone when it was prolonged for hours. Occasionally, a family member would come to pick her up and relieve her of the solitary play, but she remembered being left there often until her mother took her out of the bucket.

As she continued to narrate her story, the group members and I listened quietly. I felt a myriad of emotions including shock and sadness. My eyes visualized a toddler slipping and falling, trapped in a bucket, and my ears heard the sound of water splashing in the silence. I felt a sense of isolation when I thought that neither fun nor pain had a witness for Anita in those moments. Other members in the group shared their own experiences of shock, some cried, and a few expressed a desire to play with her. What arose in our circle was loneliness and grief. Each of us shared our experience of her story; she was moved and embarrassed by the group's responses to her narrative. I got a better understanding into her ambivalence about wanting to be seen and not seen and I said to her, 'I understand better now how stifling my time structuring could be for you [...] my attending to another person leaves you feeling unseen/unheard and when I attend to you,

DOI: 10.4324/9781003348337-7

you feel seen. Both seem overwhelming to bear?' She agreed to having mixed feelings about both experiences and told me that when my attention was on someone else in the group, she wanted to say, 'see me, look here [...] hear [...]', and when I was attentive to her, she felt 'exposed to be in the limelight'. It was a moment of connection when we sat quietly holding this quandary. At the end of that particular day, she reminded the group when it was time to close.

This change may appear to be sudden and permanent; it is not so. In the ongoing therapy group, she is still a member of, she has continued to move between frustration with the structure, which for her is a curtailment of her freedom, and her need to be connected with the group and me. The difference is that she is aware of it now, manages to catch it quickly when it happens and is able to express these frustrations. Anita's journey of awareness, healing and growth was and is incremental. The initial phase started with a love–hate relationship with me, mostly marked by persistent challenges about structure of group therapy and time. Presently, she questions me in other areas like my responses to others in the group such as, 'why are you emotionally validating this member? Why don't you challenge their behavior?' However, she is occasionally aware when she does it, and laughs while acknowledging that she wants to test my tolerance for her. The early relational experiences within the cultural context she was thrown into shaped her personality and, at times, her responses to the present environment continue to be regulated by the past.

Being a girl child in a patriarchal system in India comes with complex challenges. Socially sanctioned neglect and abuse is a norm rather than an exception. There is often an intergenerational transmission of parenting styles where the basic needs of the child go unmet. Emotional neglect and abuse are common and accepted as a way of disciplining the child and preparing her for an adult life of marriage and responsibility. Depending on class, region, religion and caste, early arranged marriages to older men is common, which the girl child is coerced into. Given these varying field conditions, it is not surprising that Anita's trust and ability to be close were compromised. What was unusual was that she had the innate capacity to challenge, rebel against and leave distressing life situations and make a life for herself. (In my experience this is not common; many girls learn to be passive and compliant to the demands of family and society.)

The fact that she challenged me was what initially drew my attention to her, which is what she wanted—to be seen. My not rejecting her combined with the other members' curiosity, admiration and liking for her perhaps helped her continue attending the group meetings. Over time, I became more cognizant of her yearning for and dread of intimacy. Between us, we co-created a movement that was marked by curiosity, excitement and an inclination to stay with the intolerable. On many occasions, she expressed in the group her interest to see where the process led her. (In fact, when I shared this chapter for feedback from her on whether I had captured her experiences accurately, I was duly chided for some of the things I had written. I had written that she was part of this group for her healing, and she corrected that saying, 'I am not here to heal, I am here for the journey'.) Over the years, we moved toward working through the challenges and talking more about the attachment we formed. All this happened in the group that was integral to Anita's journey. The other members shifted between expressing their affection for her, feeling awe at her ability to express aggression toward me, challenging her and staying with all the turmoil that would come up within the group. From her the members started learning how to express their disappointments toward me.

I was naturally inclined toward slowness, not in a hurry to get anywhere in particular with her. She moved between getting close and withdrawing. If I had become inaccessible to her when challenged repeatedly, I would have lost the opportunity for a meaningful relationship with a lovely human being. Her process of self-awareness and my inclination toward the incremental nature of healing and growth had the fortunate space and time that the group created. It is rare to have this chance of leading a group where members come back regularly over the span of many years.

In India, group therapy is usually brief given the scarcity of resources and time, and a preference for following more of a CBT or disorder-based approach. However, in my experience, awareness and change are rarely an overnight 'aha' experience; rather, it's a slow, often painful process of gaining an understanding into one's struggles. We must be aware and appreciative of the step-by-step process of therapy (Jacobs, 2017). Behavioral changes that can be sustained over time is usually an uphill task that requires intrinsic motivation and a supportive external environment. As therapists, we need to be mindful of each member's possibilities. A possibility that the therapist feels would be helpful for the member can actually be a leap into a territory which induces a high level of terror in the individual along with painful consequences.

Members in a group engage in the process of therapy when they feel some level of trust in the therapist and the group, which takes time to develop as the group goes through certain cycles of development. While keeping in mind the group processes and stages, the leader must not fall into the trap of seeing these as a given prescriptive format for all groups. Rather, therapists who follow GGT must be very mindful of preformed knowledge of groups, and labeling or pathologizing behaviors. Our theoretical knowledge about groups is indispensable; however, we must be open to immediate experience that emerges moment to moment in a group and hold all interpretations loosely.

For example, to believe that Anita was questioning the norms because it was the early stages of group development, or that she played the role of rebel in the family that resurfaced in the group would limit us from exploring further other aspects of her experience. Her experience that I am in a position of power and exercising my authority is valid because as the leader, that is part of what I do—I have collected a fee, set the group meetings and the ground rules. However democratic I may want or strive to be, I am still in a privileged position of power in the role I occupy in the group. Moreover, culturally, my role as an elder, a teacher and a therapist is often held in high esteem. Indian culture plays a part in how members interact with leaders, whether their needs and feelings are valued, as well as how they value and honor their experiences in relation to a leader. A gap in exploring all these unique factors can prove detrimental to the best possible outcomes. So, what we need to do as leaders practicing GGT is move between our theoretical understanding and the embodied experiences of the group members and ourselves.

This is where, I think, GT's phenomenological stance plays a central role in guiding the work of a GGT practitioner. GT's phenomenology is a blend of the existential phenomenology of Edmund Husserl and the experimental phenomenology of gestalt psychology (Brownell, 2016; Yontef & Jacobs, 2005). This is an adaptation of Husserl's philosophical method, which we use to pay attention to what is unfolding in our presence. Brownell (2016) says that the therapist describes what is observed rather than explaining it, and treats all observed data with equal importance without assigning value and follows the procedural dictum of observation, bracketing and description. This phenomenological work is the focus of concern for the Gestalt therapist. GT has a highly developed methodology for attending to how the therapist and patient experience each other in the therapeutic relationship. Yontef and Jacobs (2005) say that phenomenology assumes that reality is formed in the relationship between the observed and the observer, and both their subjectivities are equally valid.

Phenomenology

Phenomenology as a movement in the history of philosophy emerged in the early twentieth century in the works of Husserl, Heidegger, Sartre, Merleau-Ponty and others. Husserl was interested in the study of consciousness as experienced by the subject in his lived experience, without being influenced by theories that gave causal explanations. Phenomenology focuses on grasping various types of experience like emotion, perception, thinking, memory, embodied awareness, social awareness and linguistics (Smith, 2013). Phenomenological inquiry requires the practice of 'epoché' (a willing suspension of judgment), which is the ability to 'bracket' preconceptions, prejudices and biases—a difficult task. Gutland (2018) says that this may sound simple but it is one of the most challenging methodological requirements, because our prejudices are often blind mechanisms of judging, which we engage in passively. He goes on to add that our biases may be right or wrong, but the danger is in its blind application because if they are wrong and we do not notice them, they distort our attempts to accurately describe our experience. If we cannot accurately describe our experiences as therapists, then it certainly limits our ability to be attentive to and explore the experiences of the other in its fullness. Bracketing does not demand of us to obliterate our prejudices but instead to be conscious of them.

This methodology is useful for practicing group therapy by holding our prior knowledge flexible with an openness to what emerges in the field. The phenomenological method helps the group leader focus on each member as well as the leader's own direct experience. Although our experiences are influenced by a context that includes prior experiences, beliefs, personality functioning, culture, values and customs, we can attempt to explore how this regulates the way we make meaning of events in the present. We can further use the phenomenological attitude to reflect on what in the present situation influences our experiences and those of the group members. As in the vignette 'Colliding Subjectivities', Anita's experiences, experiences of the other group members, and mine came together to create an intersubjective field that helped us make meaning of the present event. For some members, including me, the structure created a sense of safety and control. For some, it's a source of restriction and encroachment on freedom. Over time and with support from my supervision, I was able to make meaning of our unique experiences of this situation. To explain this process further, I give below an excerpt from the conversation with my supervisor (me: VA, Supervisor: FS).

FS: How do you feel when Anita challenges you about the time frame or the way you structure the group?

VA: Well, I feel fatigued, tired especially when it keeps happening again and again [...] you know, my feelings have changed over time or rather it goes back and forth! I feel curiosity, care, love, respect, admiration [...] you know she has great chutzpah [...] however, presently I am sitting with this stuckness and feeling of frustration in my body.

FS: (laughs, I feel here a shared moment of understanding from him about my struggle as well as my mixed feelings; it's not that he states this verbally but I read this in his face.) That's a tough place to be in [...] what do you imagine will happen if you shared this with her?

(I am not describing the whole experiment in the supervision space here because I want to just capture the essence of the work rather than the whole content. I enacted a role play here of an exchange between Anita and me.)

FS: How are you feeling as you imagine sharing this with her and hearing her responses?

VA: I feel relieved in my body [...] she is connecting to what I am saying, really attentive to hearing me out. I imagine she will take it well when I share it with her in the next session.

The excerpt given above from my supervision experience is an example of exploring my phenomenology in the group as well as in the supervision space. What has often helped me in this is being able to make meaning of my feelings toward different members and the group as a whole, and my supervisor's interest has supported this work. At a structural level, I often feel confident about the framework within which I conduct groups; however, when faced with repetitive challenges I feel a bit eroded and doubtful. I also experience my space intruded upon and I want to withdraw (this is one of my enduring themes). To give you a felt sense of the group members' phenomenology in 'Colliding Subjectivities', I have provided a brief excerpt below of some of the group members.

M: I feel restless and irritated when Anita talks for too long [...] I want the sessions to wind up on time.

P: Anita, when you don't take up the time when it's offered to you and then you interrupt or want to share when someone else is sharing, elaborating on it for a long time, I start feeling disconnected [...] I lose track [...] also I want to get a break from this during the break [...]

S: Actually, you inspire me when you challenge vanaja, I wouldn't feel the courage to do so [...] not that you would not take it vanaja, but I am scared of being punished, rejected when I express disagreement or show anger. And I do feel we should take extra time if needed for closure.

R: I too feel quite inspired and brave, I wouldn't have shared my own irritation with vanaja if you hadn't done so!

N: I feel a bit scared [...] what will happen to this group if all this continues? I feel quite anxious when all this is happening and I kind of space out.

As we can see from the excerpt above, each member makes meaning of the same event in unique ways. We need to explore this in the group situation to get an accurate description of these experiences without becoming unduly influenced by our biases. To summarize Phillipson (2008), the primary task for us, while working with groups, is to maintain a phenomenological attitude, to be curious about the developing process without rushing to make meaning because meaning in this approach is multilayered, so the same event could have a different meaning for each individual, as well as the whole group.

The group leader needs to follow the principles of phenomenology to gain an understanding of how a field is organized, and through exploration see how each member experiences the field. In the context of Anita's experience, I did feel self-doubt about being too rigid about time. In the first residential retreat, I did go beyond the allocated time, which left me feeling anxiety, fatigue and shame, and from what I understood, it was overwhelming/chaotic for other group members as well as Anita, who paradoxically shared that I was not managing time well for the group. What has been helpful, over the many retreats that I have conducted, is being in touch with my felt sense, consulting my supervisor and engaging the group members in expressing their experiences.

Although I had the knowledge of how groups work and the importance of structure and boundaries, I stood firmly (sometimes shakily) on this ground. I was able to offer space for individual and cultural differences, and as a group we were able to continue in the meaning-making process of how we feel, and want to be, in communities. Fairfield (2004) says that rather than starting from an idea about how groups work and aiming at helping groups work in that way, the phenomenological approach allows us the freedom to let our theories recede into the background where they can support us. He stresses the importance of knowledge as the ground we stand on and of embracing the challenge of what we do not know and making new meanings together.

Another example I would like to share related to using a phenomenological approach that helped me navigate preformed theory and changing subjectivities was during the pandemic lockdown in March 2020. Theoretically, we know that the group goes through certain stages of development as postulated by various theoreticians. But what happens if after the establishment of cohesiveness, there is a period of chaos and fragmentation? This could happen especially in the context of a life- or world-changing event like that of the pandemic. A phenomenological attitude leads us to ask questions like, 'What is happening here? What impact does coronavirus have on an "established" group safety? What is the reason I am experiencing this group as suddenly fragmented and lost? How am I feeling, thinking and behaving in these uncertain times and how does it affect the way I relate with this group in this moment? If some members are settling down to accepting online sessions, what is happening to others? How do experiences differ from individual to individual?'

For all the members of the therapy group, the shift from in-person to online sessions was a challenge. For Anita, the feeling of frustration and anxiety was far more prolonged and intense. Although she attended all the online sessions, she usually expressed her frustration with me for not offering in-person sessions (which even if I wished to do so, I couldn't because the government had ordered a lockdown). I could have interpreted this as Anita being angry with me or avoiding contact; instead, I chose to stay with her frustrations and her underlying fear while exploring how the loss of in-person contact impacted her and other members. Although each group member expressed their anxieties related to the pandemic impact, they also expressed their anticipation for the group meetings.

One participant, who lived by herself, looked forward to this group meeting because it was an important source of succor for her in her isolation. Another member, who was a single parent, juggling her varied responsibilities, felt that the online group gave her a sense of continuity and support during the lockdown. We also talked about our experiences around dilution of time and space, feelings of interpersonal isolation that the pandemic reinforced, and frustrations with the government as a system that brought up fear and anger toward authority figures and patriarchy. As the group members shared their unique experiences, they moved from the space of COVID-19-induced physical isolation to a shared emotional togetherness. Moreover, the differences in how each member made meaning of their experiences of the same event gave Anita a different perspective, helping her become tolerant of the online format. I believe that this kind of explorative engagement provides a fulcrum that enables deeper human contact, even when external events are pulling us apart. To know that our experiences are valued is the first gift in therapy.

A phenomenological field approach would be attentive to the developmental stages and early life experiences, as well as the present field conditions that shape human experiences. I discussed earlier about how important the three foundational pillars of GT are, that is, phenomenology, field theory and dialogic existentialism. The three are interlinked, and although for the purposes of elaboration and explanation I have talked about these in separate sections, they are in reality deeply intertwined. We cannot practice one without the other, and when we do so, we are likely to fall short of capturing the whole. We cannot understand the essence of an individual's subjectivity without taking into consideration how they experience their environment, and we cannot grasp this experience without being in a meaningful dialogue that involves both the verbal and nonverbal.

The experiences of the individual group members, between members and between the leader and the group as a whole are all crucial elements. Field theory is helpful to understand Anita's ambivalence about attending online sessions. I was able to understand her irritability with me, my limitations to support her freedom, her helplessness about her freedom being curtailed, and the larger field of the sociopolitical context that the group members are a part of.

Field Theory

Field theory was developed by Lewin in the 1940s. Lewin was trained in philosophy and experimental psychology, and was greatly influenced by Gestalt theory. He borrowed the concept of field and perception from physics and Gestalt psychology and applied it to human relationships. The field theory that Lewin proposed was born in the natural sciences, specifically the theory of relativity and quantum theory that he adapted to the understanding of human behavior (Schulz, 2013). My understanding of the concept of field from a pure science perspective, is that it is an area which is under the influence of some force like electromagnetic. The field theory explains the behavior of atoms/particles and their interaction with nature. Lewin took the concept of field theory to apply it to the understanding of human behavior and developed a framework that focuses on how an individual internalizes and responds to the sociocultural environment. I think this is where it gets complex. I have personally grappled with the concept of field theory, and just when I think, 'aha, I've got this figured out', I start feeling lost again. Like Staemmler (2006) says, the attempt to apply field theory to understanding human behavior has led to a Babylonian confusion because it is difficult to comprehend the notion of the word 'field' in psychology as it requires an understanding of a new paradigm. Moreover, a number of theories have been developed around the notion of field, and for Gestalt therapists it has not been comprehensively spelled out in published writings.

Few would disagree that field theory is a core philosophical underpinning of GT, although the construct has not been well understood, discussed or applied to practice (O'Neill, 2008). Robine (2001; 2021) points out that there are a variety of ways in which people have used the term 'field theory': the organism/environment field of Perls and Goodman; the references to a background or environmental context; the Lewinian field of forces; and a phenomenological field. Although it is not easy to grasp as a concept, I appreciate the effort that's been put in by Gestalt writers like Malcolm Parlett, Jean-Marie Robine, Margherita Spagnuolo Lobb, Gary Yontef, Lynne Jacobs, Gordon Wheeler, Friedemann Schulz and Frank Staemmler to explain the concept of Gestalt therapy field theory.

I agree with Parlett (2005) and his dialogue partner Lee that the word 'field' does pose potential challenges since it can include anything and everything, is loaded with different meanings and is used interchangeably. I also see Staemmler's (2006) discomfort when he expresses how this can cause confusion and degenerate into jargon. He goes on to explain the word 'field' in its literal, extended, figurative, theoretical physics and theoretical psychology senses, before expanding on how Lewin applied the concept of field theory to understand human psychology. In fact, while reflecting on Staemmler's writing, I experienced some fear that I would obfuscate the concept of field further with my limited understanding. However, reading what Yontef (1993) has to say about field theory as the most challenging area in our conceptualization, training and practice of Gestalt therapy, was helpful. I agree with him that 'talking and reading about field theory and understanding it is very difficult, perhaps the most difficult aspect of Gestalt therapy theory to discuss' (p. 286). Furthermore, clarifying my own understanding with Friedemann Schulz was quite a comforting experience.

In addition, I do not want to abstain from explaining my understanding of field theory and its pivotal role in understanding group experiences. On a lighter note, I cannot resist the temptation to jump into the Tower of Babel,[1] speak my language and hope from this I can engage with my Gestalt community in a continued movement toward clarity, even when differences in language exist. For this purpose, I will try to focus on explaining field theory primarily based on how Lewin transferred this scientific concept to the understanding of complex human experience. Having said that, I want to acknowledge the contribution of the forefathers of GT to the incorporation of field theory in their work.

Perls was influenced by field theory, although he did not elaborate on it with the depth that Lewin did. The human being in early Gestalt therapy was conceived of as an organism–environment entity, not just an organism in an environment (Brownell, 2016). As Staemmler (2006) says, PHG (1951), when referring to the organism/environment field, were discouraging an isolationist view of human behavior. I agree with him that the intention of PHG was to point therapists toward how humankind is interlinked and argue for a movement away from the existing Cartesian divide. They emphasized how the organism and environment cannot be separated. To summarize Staemmler, human behavior has to be derived from a totality of the environment, and the varying forces in this environment are dynamic and mutually influencing. Gestalt therapy field theory is a phenomenal field theory because it's the 'perceptual experience of a certain person at a certain time, the field of any other person at any given point in time will be different, and so will the field of this person at any other point in time' (2006, p. 67).

When I use the word 'field' in the group situation, I am referring to the phenomenological field of the individuals in the group, including the therapist, their past experiences inclusive of family and culture—the subjective meaning these experiences have for them and how these mutually influence moment to moment in the group therapy situation. The individual experiences in the group cannot be separated from the environment that they takes place in, and the individual members impact the environment and each other in profound ways. We mutually co-create the emergent experiences in the whole group. As Robine (2016) says, this information gives us a wider view of the group as a 'self' that goes beyond the classical Newtonian reality of linear causality. While describing the concept of self, he says that our sense of self is unfolding, fluid, evolving, becoming by connecting through its contacts with its human and nonhuman environment. Field theory envisions the group as a whole phenomenon that carries dynamic information. I agree with him that changes in the field affect others, even in their absence and later, when members return to the group. I have observed this in the groups I conduct when a member is absent, when a new member joins or when a member leaves, over and above the sociocultural changes in each person's environment. The members in turn influence the wider social systems that they are part of outside of the group. In this sense, we are influencing and being influenced by more than our immediate environment where a greater 'whole' exists.

Human experience is so complex. There are so many forces of our past that shape our present experience, and forces in our present experience that influence our behavior as well as our envisioned experiences of our future. Having said this, it still does not capture the whole of our Gestalt. We are growing and making meaning in our environment. After we come into existence, our essence continues to develop and change in relation to one another. This is our area of work as therapists—the range of clients' and our experiences and how we influence each other. Lewin's field theory, and the advances made to it by the subsequent Gestalt thinkers, became refined in the discernment of the intersubjective processes ensuing between individuals, groups, societies and cultures.

Lewin made a profound contribution to group processes by the application of field concepts to the study of the relationship of individuals with each other and the group. Lewin postulated that human behavior is a function of the interaction between an individual and his psychological perception of the environment that together form the life space. This life space is inclusive of the person's beliefs, values, attitudes, feelings and cognitions. Gestalt psychologist Parlett (1991, 2005), talking about the importance of field and holism to understand human personality, says that for psychology to be relevant to people's experiences, therapists need to have a profound appreciation of how people live and perceive, be attentive to patterning and relationship, and recognize whole formations and complex relations—rather than slicing up nature into stimulus-response units in the manner of mechanistic science.

We can understand the person only through an understanding of the field in which they live. As Yontef and Jacobs (2005) say, a client's life story cannot tell you what actually happened in their past, but it can tell you how they experience this in the here and now field. GT views the individual's phenomenological experience within the larger environment. Although field theory and holism meaningfully influenced Perls, it was left to the later Gestalt therapists to elucidate the significance of field theory for clinical practice (Parlett, 1991, 2005; Schulz, 2013; Staemmler, 2006; Yontef, 1993). Parlett (1991) articulated this notion for GT by saying that 'the essence of field theory is that a holistic perspective towards the person extends to include environment, the social world, organizations, and culture' (p. 70). So, when I use the term 'field theory' in GGT, I am referring to the present environment of the group, how it is experienced and perceived by the members, how we influence each other, the sociocultural world we inhabit at that given moment as well as our past experiences that stimulate our present perception of the environment.

Let me illustrate this with an example for additional clarity. In one of the therapy groups that I conduct, a member named Divya, spoke about her experience of me. She described it as a force field, her yearning to be in proximity to me because it gives her a sense of protection and care, yet this need was accompanied by the need to withdraw. She shared her fear of losing this care and hopes for a continuation of it while needing to keep her distance. My own reaction to this sharing was a feeling of bewilderment, that something about me has a strong impact on her just as her reaction has on me. To understand this experience of Divya's from a holistic perspective, we need to keep in mind her past experiences of protection, safety and risk in her environment, the parents she was born to, the culture, school experiences, friendships and teachers. To understand my reaction to her, I need to be aware of my own past experiences, how I was born to a different set of parents and sociocultural events from which I derived my meaning. Added to this is our present location, loss of a parental figure for Divya and how she experiences my aging in the last few years that she has known me. My perplexity stemmed from experiencing her as independent and insulated, although I see her vulnerability and attachment to me. I also think that perhaps my own childhood experiences and the sense and aura of power I carry because of my cultural and familial experiences can be experienced as a force by some people.

Our field of experience in the present includes our perception of each other now and our past field experiences. In explaining the concept of the figure and ground dynamic, Spagnuolo Lobb and Caccamo (2013) say that the emergence of a particular experience is linked to a relational need that the client is motivated to solve. They suggest that we ask the question of how we contribute to the patient's experience at the moment and from what ground of the experience of therapeutic contact does the figure emerge for the patient. We need to engage in being curious as to why of all possible stimuli that our presence may bring, this stands out strongly for the client. Added to this, I think we need to be quite mindful of how other members experience this event. How are they influenced by what Divya says, how they individually experience me and it's bearing on the group as a whole. The relational need that the client yearns to meet is aimed toward a movement toward wholeness; it emerges from the needs of not the individual alone but also the whole group. A concept that explains this striving toward wholeness is holism, which is linked to field theory.

Holism

South African philosopher and Commonwealth statesman General Jan Smuts (1926) was the first person to use the word 'holism' in his book *Holism and Evolution*. He stated that the organism, system, universe or even the personality of an individual is not still and motionless but rather dynamic and creatively growth oriented. Smuts was influenced by the zeitgeist of his time. He was critical of Newtonian and Cartesian reductionist science and philosophy that emphasized linear causality and a fundamental split between mind and matter. He was familiar with Albert Einstein's theory of relativity and postulated that the universe was created in progressive increments. He attempted to understand the creative and complex nature of evolution and man. He proposed that there is a creative driving force that is integral to evolution, and referred to this dynamic nature as holism. Holism was the factor responsible for the progressive evolution from a simple cell to a complex organism, and finally the human personality.

The concept of holism has continued to influence many fields including biology, physics, general systems theory, anthropology, cybernetics and various branches of psychology (Wulf, 1996). Holism in the context of human development views people as inherently self-regulating and growth oriented (Schulz, 2013; Yontef & Jacobs, 2005). Holism and field theory are seen as interrelated constructs in Gestalt theory that help understand how humans move toward growth and change within the given environment—they are impacted and in turn impact the field, they grow and change in relation to the field. A client's personality and the conflicts that occur in the present can be understood in the dynamic intersubjective field in the here and now. These conflicts may stem from early experiences where the formation of a complete Gestalt was blocked; however, the evoking of these conflicts happens in relation to the present field. As one can see in 'Colliding Subjectivities', Anita's experience of being stifled was a familiar experience from childhood, yet it was evoked in the here and now by the perceived safety or the lack of it, and the meaning she derives from my actions and expressions in the present field.

Awareness into these dynamics happens over time in the therapeutic relationship, wherein the unfinished Gestalt can be addressed in the relative safety and presence of the group, which then facilitates a movement toward holism. I say relative safety because the experience of safety depends on past field conditions and what is co-created between the therapist and members. Depending on the extent of trauma or affirmation of early life space, this sense of safety can ebb and flow from moment to moment. This process is not a sudden occurrence. It is emergent, given the appropriate here-and-now field condition of safety where old trauma can be relived with interventions that support creative adjustments. The client can then steadily move toward wholeness. Once we abdicate our need to change the 'other', we can sit together in a 'safe circle' and explore new possibilities. When feelings of misunderstanding and disruptions occur, we can engage in a dialogue that can be attuned to the experiences that arise in the field.

I believe that attunement and misattunement and differing subjectivities are unavoidable in the therapeutic encounter. However, it's the ability to hold, contain and regulate these emotional states in the therapeutic bond that can help sustain the relationship and provide possibilities for repair (Atwood & Stolorow, 1984; Stolorow, 2002). There were many moments in our encounter that Anita and I experienced varying degrees of frustration with each other, just as we experienced attunement and the camaraderie of togetherness. What helped was a phenomenological attitude to look at the subjective experiences in the present field, our ability to repair the disruptions and move to the adjacent possible.

Adjacent Possible

'Adjacent Possible' is a phrase coined by the theoretical biologist Stuart Kauffman (1993, 2013, 2019) to explain evolution and biodiversity on earth. He postulated that simple cells and organisms progress into complex systems, displaying a natural order in the way they evolve. He proposes that at any given point, biological systems can only transform into more elaborate systems in certain preordained ways. He focused on the concept of self-organization, and he says that evolution of the being persistently creates its future possibilities of becoming, and what comes next in the adjacent possible, emerges from what is here and now—the actual.

Kauffman's theory has been applied to many fields including biology, technology, creative innovations in organizations, and cultural evolution to understand and explain progress in general. Adjacent possible can be described as any phenomenon, whether physical, social or historical, interacting with other phenomena and it changes in relation to the other. It's a biological possibility that growth and change happen in a natural and relational manner. Applying this concept to human personality and their responses to developmental yearnings, we often observe that human development is incremental as well.

The concept of adjacent possible has been explained with an example in chapter 5 of this book. Steven Johnson (2010) describes adjacent possible beautifully as he applies the concept to innovation, saying that the adjacent possible is a kind of shadow future, which hovers on the edge of the present and its boundaries grow as you explore them—like opening a door that leads to the possibility of a new door. An infant has to first learn how to crawl before she can start walking. Any attempts to speed up the process of development can lead to trauma. Patience and stillness can lead to each minute step opening up new possibilities in the developmental milestones. In relational GT, we apply this concept to understand human personality development and change (L. Jacobs, personal communication, 2017). An emergent Gestalt that is figural and dealt with can lay the groundwork for another figure forming, thus creating novel opportunities for the next adjacent possible.

When we combine phenomenology, field theory and holism with Kauffman's adjacent possible, we can be attentive to clients as well as to our experiences—past, and present, organismic yearning for integration and growth, and the incremental and inevitable nature of change. I believe that each relational moment in therapy is an opportunity for future possibilities as well as a gradual movement toward wholeness. When we look at an individual, a group or an organization, we can perceive a whole—like the individual in the group. Yet, the individual is a part in relation with other 'wholes' in the larger field.

As we expand this concept of 'part' and 'whole', we can see that the group is part of larger systems like family, culture, society and political situation. Every whole we perceive is part of a larger whole in the field, 'a field is a systematic web of relationships and exists in a context of even larger webs of relationships' (Yontef, 1993, p. 298). When we apply these concepts to group dynamics, then the implication is that the members in the group are interacting with the leader, with each other, identifying their organismic needs, regulating these in relation to the environment, and finding resolutions to meet these in the best possible manner.

Application of these theoretical constructs help us understand how individual group members develop awareness, growth and change and how this impacts the group as a whole. It suggests that Herculean ideas and major changes cannot be reached until we explore the tiny possibilities in between. I never have an idea of what will ultimately happen in the group, and I believe that whatever will happen is what is within the possibility of that group. I am at peace with that. To be honest, I enjoy the process like I used to when I played hopscotch with my brother—challenge, frustration, excitement and play.

I will share an example to illuminate the importance of staying with the group's process and adjacent possible, as opposed to pushing for an agenda stemming out of our own personal expectations as leaders. Many years ago, I was requested by an organization to facilitate a group of educators who were in a six-month residential training program to develop basic skills in counseling adolescents. I was one of the external faculty members involved in the teaching. Toward the latter half of this program, the director of the center requested that I conduct a week-long group therapy for the trainees, focusing on awareness and growth. The director was present for the first morning half of the group meeting. He started to get anxious when, after the initial ice breaker activity, the members hesitantly shared their expressive artwork before drifting off into what seemed like an awkward silence just before the tea break. We all sat there for a few minutes in the stillness. To my personal discomfiture, the director started to remonstrate with the group to work with me, telling them how valuable my time was. I was concerned about this approach, so I suggested we break for tea and I took him aside and explored the source of his fears. Since we had known each other for many years and we shared a fairly trusting relationship, it was easy for me to explain to him how expecting the members to jump in and work with me might be a tad unrealistic. I requested him to trust the process enough to leave the room and await what would unfold.

When we resumed post tea, I checked in with the group members about their experiences of safety in the group, and invited them to share at their pace and comfort. I shared my own early experiences of being in groups where I had concerns around safety, acceptance and confidentiality. Some members came forward to share their fears and concerns. It was after the lunch break that one member of the group shared his experience in one of the training classes with this group. He had an unpleasant experience of his personal sharing in the class, being informally brought up outside the class by another member, which left him feeling ashamed. The person who unwittingly broke the confidentiality apologized. After this event, other members started opening up, sharing their experiences from childhood related to trust and safety. Some members shared their experiences of shame during adolescence, in their developing sexuality and gender identities in the school and home environment. This process was not in any way preplanned, and when I used the expressive art activity in the beginning of the group process, I had no idea that it would take this trajectory.

A week later when the group came to an end, most members had shared, gained awareness and worked on some of their painful struggles with authority figures and ideas around sexuality. Moreover, they developed an awareness into how their adolescent experiences had impacted the way they dealt with their own students. Some were able to treat their students with tolerance and some shared how they unwittingly came down harshly on their students. A common theme that emerged was the attitude toward developing sexuality during adolescence, how it was dealt with by teachers, and the cultural differences in the way girls and boys were expected to behave.

The conditioning around maintaining distance between the sexes during puberty is quite high in India. Sexuality and expressions of sexual interest are restricted, and going against this norm results in public shaming and at times punishment. Adolescent behavior is shaped in this social environment, and the individual internalizes a psychological understanding of this experience. Sadly, this is accompanied with the potential harm to their adult sexual life as well as interpersonal interactions. Many of the teachers shared how they restricted girls from interacting with boys in their work setting. When asked about their experiences of first crushes and infatuations during their teenage years, many of them recollected experiences that evoked shame as well as innocent joy. They had been reprimanded by their parents and teachers for their developing sexuality, yet internally there was a joy at recollecting the excitement of a first crush.

The adjacent possible for the members of this group was creating an awareness around how their school experiences had shaped their own ideas around sexuality, and the cultural shaming that accompanied a normative developmental stage. It also offered a possibility of building a narrative for how they would want to be different as teachers, and be mindful of social shaming. Understanding how the individual's behavior is a function of their internalizations and sociocultural influences is vital for working with individuals and groups. Engaging together in a mindful process, clarifying the normalcy of developmental stages and experiences, and sharing narratives with different perspectives within the safe circle can facilitate meaning making and belongingness.

Note

1 The Tower of Babel narrative in Genesis 11:1–9 tells how the Babylonians wanted to make a name for themselves by building a tower that aimed to reach the heavens. This was disrupted by God by confusing the language of the workers so that they could no longer understand one another.

References

Atwood, G. E., & Stolorow, R. D. (1984). *Structures of subjectivity: Explorations in psychoanalytic phenomenology.* Analytic Press.

Brownell, P. (2016). Contemporary gestalt therapy. In D. J. Cain, K. Keenan, & S. Rubin (Eds.), *Humanistic psychotherapies: Handbook of research and practice* (pp. 219–250). American Psychological Association.

Fairfield, M. A. (2004). Gestalt groups revisited: A phenomenological approach. *Gestalt Review, 8*(3), 336–357. https://doi.org/10.5325/gestaltreview.8.3.0336

Gutland, C. (2018). Husserlian phenomenology as a kind of introspection. *Frontiers in Psychology, 9*, 896. https://doi.org/10.3389/fpsyg.2018.00896

Jacobs, L. (2017). Hopes, fears, and enduring relational themes. *British Gestalt Journal, 26*(1), 7–16.

Johnson, S. (2010, September 25). *The genius of the tinkerer. Wall Street Journal.* www.wsj.com/articles/SB10001424052748703989304575503730101860838.

Kauffman, S. (2013, March 22). *Beyond reductionism twice: No laws entail biosphere evolution, formal cause laws beyond efficient cause laws.* arXiv.org. https://doi.org/10.48550/arXiv.1303.5684

Kauffman, S. (2019). Innovation and the evolution of the economic web. *Entropy, 21*(9), 864. https://doi.org/10.3390/e21090864

Kauffman, S. A. (1993). *The origins of order: Self-organization and selection in evolution.* Oxford University Press.

O'Neill, B. (2008). Relativistic quantum field theory: Implications for gestalt therapy. *Gestalt Review, 12*(1), 7–23. https://doi.org/10.5325/gestaltreview.12.1.0007

Parlett, M. (1991). Reflections on field theory. *British Gestalt Journal, 1*, 68–91. www.elementsuk.com/libraryofarticles/fieldtheory.pdf.

Parlett, M., & Lee, R. (2005). Contemporary gestalt therapy: Field theory. In A. L. Woldt & S. M. Toman (Eds.), *Gestalt therapy: History, theory, and practice* (pp. 41–64). SAGE.

Perls, F. S. (1969). *Ego, hunger and aggression: The beginning of gestalt therapy.* Vintage/Random House.

Perls, F. S., Goodman, P., & Hefferline, R. F. (1951). *Gestalt therapy: Excitement and growth in the human personality.* Dell.

Phillipson, P. (2008). A gestalt theory of group psychotherapy. In B. Feder & J. Frew (Eds.), *Beyond the hot seat revisited: Gestalt approaches to group* (pp. 39–51). Gestalt Institute Press.

Robine, J.-M. (2001). From field to situation. In J.-M. Robine (Ed.), *Contact and relationship in a field perspective* (pp. 95–107). L'Exprimerie.

Robine, J.-M. (2016). *Self: Une polyphonie de gestalt-thérapeutes contemporains.* L'Exprimerie.

Robine, J.-M. (2021). On the good use of incohérence. *Gestalt Review, 25*(2), 161–177. https://doi.org/10.5325/gestaltreview.25.2.0161

Schulz, F. (2013). Roots and shoots of gestalt therapy field theory: Historical and theoretical developments. *Gestalt Journal of Australia and New Zealand, 10*(1), 24–47.

Smith, D. W. (2013, December 16). *Phenomenology. Stanford Encyclopedia of Philosophy.* https://plato.stanford.edu/entries/phenomenology/

Smuts, J. C. (1926). *Holism and evolution.* Macmillan.

Spagnuolo Lobb, M., & Caccamo, J. (2013). The now-for-next in group psychotherapy: The magic of staying together. *Cahiers de Gestalt-Therapy, 1*(2), 25–38. https://doi.org/10.3917/cges.ns01.0025

Staemmler, F. (2006). A Babylonian confusion?: On the uses and meanings of the term field. *British Gestalt Journal, 15*(2), 64–83. www.bowmancounseling.com/wp-cont ent/uploads/2018/05/Staemmler-on-FIeld-Theory-1.pdf.

Stolorow, R. D. (2002). From drive to affectivity: Contextualizing psychological life. *Psychoanalytic Inquiry, 22*(5), 678–685. https://doi.org/10.1080/07351692209349012

Wulf, R. (1996). The historical roots of gestalt therapy theory. *Gestalt Dialogue: Newsletter for the Integrative Gestalt Centre.* www.gestalt.org/wulf.htm.

Yontef, G. M. (1993). *Awareness, dialogue & process: Essays on gestalt therapy.* Gestalt Journal Press.

Yontef, G., & Jacobs, L. (2005). Gestalt therapy. In R. J. Corsini & D. Wedding (Eds.), *Current psychotherapies* (pp. 342–380). Thomson Brooks/Cole.

Chapter 7

Martin Buber's Dialogic Existentialism

Disruptions and Dialogue

*Pari (a female participant in her 30s) and Vinay (a male participant in his 30s)
were part of an ongoing therapy group that I conducted some years ago. Pari
was helpful by nature and had been supportive of Vinay during his academic
and professional struggles in the early years of their courtship. However, over
time conflicts started cropping up in their relationship. From early childhood,
Pari had been conditioned to not express her disappointments directly and held
them in a tight rein. She would feel helpless each time she experienced a lack of
recognition for her caring and wished to be acknowledged for the support she
extended to Vinay. He was an easygoing partner and yearned for nurturance,
while feeling smothered when he experienced it. He responded to this feeling of
overwhelm through anger or withdrawal. While being part of the group, their
relationship went through a severe conflict, ending in hurtful exchanges and a
breakup. Both were left with feelings of shock, hurt, anger and shame. This had
an impact on each of them individually, their relationship with each other and
the group as a whole. We were all sitting in what felt like a co-created 'minefield' with feelings of self-doubt, apprehension, anxiety, isolation and hope.
I was concerned that if these profound feelings that I sensed did not find a space
to be explored and expressed, it would leave the group members in a state of
unprocessed confusion. Moreover, two people at least would feel unmet in their
deep sense of isolation.*

*They decided to share their discomfort rather than drop out or be emotionally
checked out from the group. As they shared their subjective narratives, I sensed
Pari's shock, anxiety and shame—shock because this was the first time that
she had experienced such a painful fight, anger at being attacked, and shame
at her uncontrolled anger directed at him. I had a felt sense of Vinay's shock,
anger, and shame—shock at the way the fight escalated to its terrible end, anger
at self and Pari for the violent exchanges, and shame about his volatility. This
was compounded by the shame both experienced talking about it in the group.
I explored their feelings after their sharing, and the feelings of the other group
members, before inviting them to communicate with each other directly.*

DOI: 10.4324/9781003348337-8

I requested their permission to regulate their sharing, especially if I had an idea about a different response to how they usually communicated with each other during arguments. I suggested that they listen while the other shared and reflect back only the feelings behind the sharing. I interrupted each time I observed either of them getting defensive with the other or accusing the other for being insensitive, and asked them to observe how they felt when they converted their statements into 'You felt shamed when I said insensitive things about your femininity', 'You felt shocked and rejected when I slapped you and asked you to leave'. Although most of the group members and I could imagine and reflect on how both of them felt, Pari and Vinay found it very challenging to own their feelings, take responsibility for their reactions and imagine the other's experience. I think this is quite common in couple relationships when each person feels that they have been hurt by the other and emotions are running high. It's difficult to feel empathic.

Yet, the process was completed where they got the chance to talk and listen, and the group members were invited to share their experiences. The group members got in touch with their own struggles in intimate relationships and difficulty in practicing empathy when one is angry with the partner. This work became possible because the group members had been together for more than a year (and in individual therapy with their respective therapists for three to four years), and there was a sufficient level of trust, mutual care and willingness to be honest. In addition, both Pari and Vinay were quite reflective and committed to the journey of personal awareness and change. They continued to communicate with each other in the following sessions, hoping to find some healing through their verbal exchanges. Their attempts toward honesty with each other and appreciation of how each one subjectively experienced this fight, facilitated the possibility of new ways of relating over a period of time.

Every moment of meeting between the group members and between the leader and members is a moment of meaningful contact of universality and the uniqueness of human existence. I think the group setting provides a larger context than individual therapy to explore the polarities of human anxieties like intimacy and isolation, agency and thrownness. It also gives us the opportunity to see how each of us relates subjectively to these existential dilemmas, thus co-creating a space of awareness, learning and growth. Developing the ability to genuinely meet each other in their subjective spaces, while appreciating the differences, facilitates the development and establishment of healthy connections. The members can take these new ways of relating with the self and the other into their lived spaces in the world outside.

This natural rhythm and the language to know and express what we need and want in a relationship develops in early relationships—early caregivers, family, school, community and our cultural context. The closest way to describe this 'knowing' how to be in a relational process can be termed as what Lyons-Ruth et al. (1998) and Lyons-Ruth (1999, 2007) call 'procedural' or 'relational knowing'.[1] As children, we learn how to express our feelings, thoughts and desires, and the language in which we express this is learned in relation to the other. Both Pari and Vinay developed their creative ways of expressing their needs in their early environment; however, these had become cemented over the years. Their expression of genuine feelings was blocked, because the expression of their real feelings was systemically impermissible in their early relational field. For example, as a girl Pari experienced a confusing version of feminine and masculine in relation to her mother and other women in the household, marked by the absence of a significant male figure. She witnessed a helpless, hopeless and voiceless side that would switch to an aggressive side on occasions when feeling cornered. Vinay experienced his mother as switching between aggression and helplessness, and his father as withdrawn and aggressive, both as a recipient of this behavior as well as a witness to how his father and mother related with each other. These patterns got shaken when both of them tried to practice talking to each other in a different manner than what they were accustomed to. They engaged in trying to communicate their real feelings to each other, thereby facilitating an awareness into their set ways of relating that no longer worked in adult relationships. This is an important step in a relational situation and what can follow is the strengthening of procedural knowing, of how to express themselves, and learning to meet each other in an authentic manner that is not colored by their childhood history.

For them, practicing genuine communication, listening and confirming each other without interruptions and bringing their real vulnerable feelings into the relational field helped heighten the quality of contact. This also helped the other group members gain a deeper understanding into how each of them moved between the polarity of intimacy and isolation. They got an opportunity to be mindful of how one's perception and expressions about self, others and the world are formed in early relationships and how these can be reformed and expressed in a manner that is open to genuine dialogue. Through experience and observation, they got an understanding into how human yearning for intimacy is unconsciously avoided through a monologue that negates the subjective experience of the other. I believe, both had a shame detoxification experience in the group setting, which may have been probably more isolating in individual therapy because acceptance and individual sharing from group members have a unique power to correct relational trauma in contrast to feedback from one lone therapist.

Every individual being is part of a larger cosmos of relationships, and the group is a representation of the interconnected and relational nature of this universe. At the heart of this universe is the human ability to engage in a dialogue, as defined by Buber, to make contact, meaning and human relatedness. Buber is considered one of the most important existential philosophers of the twentieth century. He influenced philosophy, religion, education and psychotherapy—in particular GT (Buber, 1991; Buber & Buber, 1999; Hycner, 1993, 1995; Hycner & Jacobs, 1995; Martin, 2017; Schulz, 2004;

Watson, 2006; Yontef & Jacobs, 2005). While living in Germany, and later in Palestine, Buber promoted a philosophy for healing and change through the practice of dialogue. GT rests on an approach toward human existence that is phenomenological field in its theory and dialogic in its methodology in the therapeutic relationship.

The dialogic relationship is ideal for the kind of curative connection that is aligned with the Gestalt concept of change. A GT therapist who functions from a dialogic position will establish a here and now, contactful and non-judgmental dialogue that encourages the client to deepen awareness. Only through acceptance of how we are at the given moment can change emerge—rejection of self is counterintuitive to change.

Dialogic Existentialism

Buber was a Hasidic scholar and his idea concerning dialogue was built on the Jewish tradition, which believes that a dialogic engagement with the other is equivalent to engaging in dialogue with God (Jacobs, 1998). While explaining Buber's philosophy Jacobs says that Buber was interested in human experience and believed that human beings cannot be known as objects in the world, that we need to have a dialogue with them as subjects, to understand how they make meaning of their existence. In his *Tales of the Hasidim* (1991), Buber specified three kinds of dialogue (as cited by Morgan, 2007). Morgan has described these three kinds of dialogues specified by Buber as genuine, technical and monologue. Genuine dialogue can be spoken or silent, where the therapist is attuned to the client with a commitment toward inclusion. Technical dialogue is procedural and is intended for an understanding of clients presenting concerns, for example, the process of a semistructured interview to get conceptual clarity into the client's problem. Monologue is when we talk at the client in a tangential way that misses a true meeting of two subjects. Monologue avoids togetherness and keeps both client and therapist in isolation in the therapeutic relationship. According to Buber, only genuine dialogue has the power to establish a relational connection through which healing and change are possible.

Dialogue can be further elucidated through Buber's description of two modes of relating—'I-Thou' and 'I-It'—which are the two relational orientations of meeting the other. Buber defined the authentic meeting between two persons as the I-Thou relationship, and emphasized this genuine dialogue as the most important aspect of human experience (Hycner, 1993, 1995; Hycner & Jacobs, 1995; Yontef, 1993; Yontef & Fairfield, 2008). In an I-Thou relationship, the personal relationship is at the center of attention. This refers to an approach of being with another person that Buber says is an end in itself and a healing through meeting (Jacobs, 1991, 1998; Schulz, 2004). According to Schulz (2004), fundamental to Buber's idea of healing through meeting is the belief that the therapeutic relationship is a holographic picture of relational dynamics in the patient's life, and that relational changes in the therapeutic relationship will affect the patient's other relational events. Buber contrasted this I-Thou relationship with an I-It relationship, where the relationship is at the periphery and the main focus is to get certain needs, functions and tasks met. Pointing out the difference in modes of relating between human and natural sciences, Schulz (2004) says that in human sciences, the I-Thou mode is predominant and in natural sciences, the I-It mode dominates. We are not fully human if we cannot relate in an I-Thou mode. At the same time, I-It is an important mode of relating interpersonally to be able to meet our needs in a healthy way. In a therapeutic relationship, assessment, diagnosis and interventions will have an I-It and an I-Thou mode to them. For example, if a therapist does an empty chair because it makes them feel good, then it's an I-It mode. If a therapist is not so concerned about how they appear to the client and waits until the experiment feels needed or possible out of caring for the client, then it's an I-Thou mode. In the dialogic attitude, the therapist is present to an I-Thou mode of relating, where the client is met in their lived space of phenomenology. Buber contended that both modes of relating are necessary for living and that in trying to meet our clients as best as we can, we are flowing in and out of being with them, thinking, being in touch with feelings and interacting moment to moment.

As compared to dialogue, monologue can be looked at as a mode of relating where the ability to see the other as a valid presence with a separate identity is missing. I believe that monologue is an important stage of development in early infancy, and it may also present itself in the way client and therapist relate with each other. This is likely to happen if early relational experiences have been marked by meager or limited meeting in the relational matrix. The therapist staying in monologue mode is risky for the client's well-being. This can happen when we are focused on meeting our own narcissistic needs for validation and mirroring from the client. This can also occur when we feel nervous/inadequate as a therapist and want to educate the client or talk to the client without an engagement. Sometimes monologue is important, for example when we give a lecture, although, when I am giving a lecture to my students, I still want to meet them with a dialogic attitude, not just talk to them but really connect with how they experience what I am saying. 'Nothing is pure, monologue or dialogue, we keep moving between different modes' (F. Schulz, personal communication, 2021).

In the story narrated above, my felt sense of what Pari and Vinay were feeling, my care for them and my exploring and reflecting that to them would be the I-Thou mode. My assessment that the group was sitting in a 'minefield', suggesting an experiment and alternate responses, would move into an I-It mode. When they were attentive to the pain felt by the other, and acknowledged that, it would be the I-Thou mode between the couple. Healthy relationship requires flexibility and a natural rhythm that can move between the I-Thou and I-It modes of relating (Hycner & Jacobs,1995; Yontef & Schulz, 2016).

In the last four decades or so, some schools of psychotherapy have been moving toward a worldview that incorporates Buber's philosophy of dialogue into their practice. According to Jacobs (1991), many of these theories do not acknowledge Buber's philosophy, but it is part of a general 'Weltanschauung'[2] that affects the development of new ideas in psychology. The intersubjective theorists (Orange, 2009; Orange, Atwood, & Stolorow, 1999; Stolorow, 2002; Stolorow, 2008; Stolorow, Brandchaft, & Atwood, 2014) have introduced Buber's philosophy of dialogue into psychoanalytic thinking, thus causing analytic work to move from a one-person intrapsychic exploration to a dyadic interpersonal model. GT from its inception clearly rested on Buber's philosophy; however, the emphasis on the criticality of dialogue is something that has grown in the last few decades with relational GT and it is the only therapy that places Buber's philosophy as the cornerstone of its therapeutic practice (Hycner, 1993, 1995; Jacobs, 1998; Schulz, 2004; Yontef, 1993). Expanding his philosophical premise of these modes of relating and dialogue, Buber postulated three fundamental components of dialogic existentialism, which are inclusion, presence and commitment to dialogue.

Inclusion

Buber (1965) indicated in his writings how the psychotherapist, like the educator or anyone who wants to establish a genuine dialogical relationship, needs to practice inclusion. He described inclusion as 'a bold swinging demanding the most intensive stirring of one's being into the life of the other' (p. 81, as cited in Hycner & Jacobs, 1995). It's trying to feel with our body and mind what the client must be experiencing. This is somewhat similar to Rogerian empathy, where one imagines the felt experience of the other. However, for Buber empathy did not capture the essence of inclusion because inclusion acknowledges both poles of relationality, that is, the therapist being attuned to the client's experience as well as to the therapist's own (Buber & Buber, 1999). It necessitates entering the world of the client accompanied by an embodied experience of what they are feeling, sensing and thinking. This happens in tandem with the process of being able to retain one's own separate sense of self; otherwise, this process can lead to confluence, which does not recognize the distinct separateness of self and other.

In a group that I conducted a few years ago, I remember a 40-year-old woman, Ahalya, who expressed how life is a series of compromises and sacrifices and, ultimately, we are left with nothing at the end except bitter disillusionment. She ended this sharing by turning to me and saying, 'don't you agree?' I was startled by the suddenness of the question addressed to me and asked her if she was asking for my personal opinion of whether I experienced my life similarly. She responded with, 'yes, of course'. I responded to her with, 'I do want to answer your question, and before that I wanted to say that it's painful for you to sit here, look back at your life and see all the sacrifices you have made, I wonder how you feel?' She continued with expressing her anger, resentment and loss of identity. Toward the end of the explorations and reflections, I said to her, 'yes, I see where you are in this moment feeling regret, pain and anger at the loss of your dreams, yes I have had my share of compromises, loss of dreams and regrets [...] no I don't agree that there's nothing left at the end for me [...] how does this land on you?' Ahalya responded by saying that she appreciated my honesty in sharing my thoughts rather than trying to agree or deny her experiences wholeheartedly.

Through imagining and communicating the client's experience, the therapist validates the existence of the client and self who share a universal existential affinity and yet have their unique individual feelings. Hycner and Jacobs (1995) define inclusion as the 'back-and-forth movement' of being able to go over to the 'other side' and yet remain centered in one's own existence (p. 20). This requires the therapist to have a strong sense of their own centeredness while being able to be psychologically flexible to feel the client's experience. This can be fairly daunting for us because it requires being human and allowing ourselves to be touched by the client. This process of practicing inclusion with the client is one-sided, as in, the therapist understands the client's world but cannot expect the client to understand the therapist's world (Jacobs, 1989; Yontef, 1993; Hycner, 1993). If we expect inclusion from our clients, then it is no longer a client–therapist relationship and it has probably moved into a friendship, which is reciprocal.

Presence

In inclusion, we try to get close to the client's experiences, and in presence we are in touch with our experiences. Thus, we can see that inclusion and presence are intertwined, and the example I gave above of Ahalya reflects this interconnection. Presence is based on the idea that true meeting can only happen when there is a transparent engagement with the client without the need to hide behind a mask that claims objectivity or neutrality. If the client can witness the therapist without the mask of imperviousness, they may be able to risk their vulnerable self while accepting the limitations of being human. Presence, I think, is akin to the Rogerian concept of congruence and self-disclosure. This involves a strong sense of self-acceptance with which the therapist allows self to be seen as they are with their vulnerabilities, strengths, limitations, perceptions and feelings. Jacobs says that presence is the ability to let go of all technical concerns and goals and bring one's true being into the dialogue. 'Being' involves bringing one's authentic self into the therapy room, and 'seeming' involves bringing what one believes others will approve of (Hycner & Jacobs, 1995; Martin, 2017). They say that inauthentic ways of relating destroy the possibility of an I-Thou relationship. They talk about presence as the most rudimentary element yet the most difficult to practice because we may wish to be seen and be validated as a good therapist by the client. I think overvaulting ambition to be seen as an expert therapist, can also lead to disproportionate shame when we receive severe criticism as a 'bad therapist', which can result in disruptions in contact and probably a shift into monologue. I agree with Cole (2013) that a holistic view of our self, which includes an acceptance of our shadowed parts, is very important for us to ensure that we don't abuse our power as group leaders. Although presence is challenging as therapists, we need to take the time to reflect and explore what our struggles are in being congruent, in order to develop the ability to be present. However, it is important to keep in mind that presence requires an ability to navigate between being congruent and harmful self-disclosure. Although Buber believed that dialogue requires unreserved communication, we must keep in mind that as therapists this is not fully possible. We need to filter as per the need of the clinical situation. As Spagnuolo Lobb and Wheeler (2013) say, it's a real encounter between two people that is unique and in which the reciprocal perceptions are modified and the patterns of the past are developed with a view to improving this relationship, not that of the past.

Generally, in groups I facilitate, I share how I experience individual members as well as the group. I also disclose my life experiences when I feel that I resonate with someone's sharing of their pain. However, I exercise caution because I believe that the therapist needs to be attuned to the ability of the member to tolerate this disclosure. There needs to be a sensitivity to how disclosure will impact the particular member and the whole group, and it's important to moderate it depending on the stage the group is in, the extent of cohesiveness, the therapeutic bond with the leader and also the resilience of each individual member to tolerate it. Jacobs says that it does not involve a willy-nilly sharing of one's full self. One needs to modulate how much of one's self can be brought in based on the stage of therapy and the need of each individual client.

I agree with her and I have experienced this in person as a member of the PGI residential group. I remember narrating a traumatic event from childhood that left me emotionally vulnerable, and the group leader disclosed an experience of their own that had similar nuances and checked with me wondering if their sharing was intrusive. I believe this willingness of the leader to be vulnerable in the group with me and explore how this impacted me helped foster a sense of being seen and understood.

Commitment to Dialogue

Dialogue is unpredictable and a commitment to it means that as a therapist I cannot be invested in a particular outcome. It implies that we are devoted to staying with the client's experience, even if we cannot understand it. According to Schulz (2004), commitment to dialogue is a form of relating that is based on what the client and therapist experience in relation to the other, and the therapist's willingness and curiosity to comprehend this experience with an ongoing engagement. The therapist approaches the therapeutic task with the attitude that clients' and one's own phenomenological experience is equally valid and true. The dialogue, that is, the in-between space created by the therapist and client in the I-Thou mode, is the healing element and not the therapist (Hycner, 1993, 1995; Hycner & Jacobs, 1995; Schulz, 2004; Yontef, 1993). Hycner (1995), in explaining this, says that Buber calls this the between space, referring to the quality of dialogue that is larger than the sum of two people talking. Neither the therapist nor the client can control the outcome of dialogue. In fact, both have to surrender to the emergent phenomena from this co-created field. Yontef (1993) says that dialogue is not a process of forcing one's singular preconceived ideas of what is best for the client, nor is it following the client's narratives blindly and negating one's own experience. It's an ability to walk between the two psychological realms carefully and bring to the foreground what emerges in the indeterminate space. He says that in a genuine dialogue, both sides have valuable and needed perspectives to contribute. The therapist's job is to be invested in exploring these perspectives and a shared understanding, and the unique differences are an equally important aspect of acknowledging the human condition.

In dialogical theory, the therapist is responsible for consistently maintaining an attitude of genuine dialogue; however, the agency of the client is given equal primacy and it is the client who will ultimately choose to participate in the process of dialogue. Thus, dialogical therapy brings a serious emphasis on existential responsibility for both the therapist and client. Yontef (1993) says that in the dialogic attitude, the therapist makes himself available to an I-Thou relating, which does not mean that we are always nice to each other but show genuine caring through honesty, rather than continual softness.

Application to Groups

Dialogical existentialism in GT is a robust relational approach to understanding an individual's relationship with self and others, to the family, society and the universe at large. Hycner (1993, 1995) says that it places the development of individual and pathology within the interconnected tapestry of systems that form and reform the expression of the intrapsychic, interpersonal and transpersonal realm. The fundamental principles of Buber's philosophy accommodate with ease to its application to group therapy. Groups, as shared earlier, are a microcosm of the individual's world outside, while also being a creative space for forging new ways of relating to the world. In a group setting, the members are directly and indirectly in contact with each other, thus providing an opportunity to gain awareness into the way each individual establishes or refrains from contact. Given the right field condition of inclusion, presence and dialogue facilitated by the group leader, the members can experiment with creative ways of contacting the self and the other.

Relevance to Indian Cultural Context

As highlighted in chapter 3, research findings and psychotherapy practice in Indian culture highlight certain common characteristics of Indian culture that separate it from Western culture. In the story narrated above, it was important for me to be able to experience an approximation of both Pari's and Vinay's thoughts, feelings and beliefs. It was also crucial to have a working knowledge of the cultural context and its impact on their respective intrapsychic world. Indian womanhood is shaped within a gendered hierarchy, where submissiveness, purity, gentleness and nurturance are deified, and aggression, assertion, ambition and overt expressions of sexuality are discouraged and disapproved of. Indian women are struggling to deconstruct personal identities entrenched in patriarchal norms and reconstruct a selfhood based on what is meaningful and true for them (Guzder & Krishna, 2005; Guzder et al., 2014). However, emancipation from internalized patriarchy and confidence about one's own identity is a distant dream for many of us. Similarly, Indian manhood has also been shaped in the sociocultural field of patriarchy and ascribed feminine and masculine roles. During infancy and early childhood, the male child is often celebrated, smothered and revered. Yet, as the Kakar (2012) and Kakar and Kakar (2007) say, as the male child moves toward adolescence, there is often an unexpected withdrawal of unconditional maternal nurturance accompanied with expressive expectations to become strong, brave, ambitious and productive. Indians in general search for relational connectedness, belongingness, dependency and interdependence in their relationships as opposed to autonomy and independence. In a therapeutic context, this need is more pervasive, and I think Buber's dialogic existentialism embedded in relationality can have a natural appeal in our cultural setting.

Interdependence is a phenomenon that develops over time in the later phases of adult life among many Indians, and dependence is both fostered and encouraged late into adult life. I think a purely Western classical therapeutic stance that associates mental health with autonomy, individuation from family systems, and agency to exercise one's freedom are unlikely to resonate well with the Indian ethos. However, GT's therapeutic relationship, which is founded on the concept of Buber's dialogic existentialism, can be easily assimilated into our work. Given the Jewish tradition from which Buber evolved his theory, which is respectful of the 'otherness' and appreciative of human existential needs for connectedness, the fundamental principles of dialogic existentialism have a synchronicity to Indian culture. A dialogically informed psychotherapy practice, grounded in the phenomenological field, helps us make meaning of our client experiences and learn from them about their culture, how they have been shaped by these and how they are impacted in the here and now.

Notes

1   How to be in a relationship, how to relate with intimate others
2   Weltanschauung: A particular worldview

References

Atwood, G. E., & Stolorow, R. D. (1984). *Structures of subjectivity: Explorations in psychoanalytic phenomenology*. Analytic Press.

Buber, M. (1965). *The knowledge of man: A philosophy of the interhuman. Selected essays*. (M. S. Friedman, Ed.). Harper & Row.

Buber, M. (1991). *Tales of the Hasidim*. Schocken Books.

Buber, M., & Agassi, J. B. (1999). *Martin Buber on psychology and psychotherapy: Essays, letters, and dialogue*. Syracuse University Press.

Cole, P. (2013). In the shadow of the leader: Power, reflection, and dialogue in gestalt group therapy. *Gestalt Review, 17*(2), 178–189. https://doi.org/10.5325/gestaltreview.17.2.0178

Guzder, J., & Krishna, M. (2005). Sita-Shakti @ cultural collision: Issues in the psychotherapy of diaspora Indian women. In S. Akhtar (Ed.), *Freud along the Ganges: Psychoanalytic reflections on the people and culture of India* (pp. 205–233). Other Press.

Guzder, J., Santhanam-Martin, R., & Rousseau, C. (2014). Gender, power and ethnicity in cultural consultation. In L. J. Kirmayer, J. Guzder, & Cécile Rousseau (Eds.), *Cultural consultation: Encountering the other in mental health care* (pp. 163–182). Springer.

Hycner, R. (1993). *Between person and person: Toward a dialogical psychotherapy*. Gestalt Journal Press.

Hycner, R. (1995). The dialogic ground. In L. R. Jacobs & R. Hycner (Eds.), *Healing relationship in gestalt therapy: A dialogic-self psychology approach* (pp. 55–66). Gestalt Journal Press.

Hycner, R., & Jacobs, L. R. (1995). *Healing relationship in gestalt therapy: A dialogic-self psychology approach*. Gestalt Journal Press.

Jacobs, L. (1989). Dialogue in gestalt theory and therapy. *Gestalt Journal, 12*(1), 25–67.

Jacobs, L. (1991, October). *The therapist as 'other:' The patient's search for relatedness* [Conference presentation]. Martin Buber's contribution to the humanities. https://secureservercdn.net/50.62.174.80/y1a.e81.myftpupload.com/wp-content/uploads/2021/09/therapist_asothers.pdf.

Jacobs, L. (1998, March). *Dialogue and paradox* [Lecture-discussion transcript]. Captured at the Portland Gestalt Therapy Training Institute. https://secureservercdn.net/50.62.174.80/y1a.e81.myftpupload.com/wp-content/uploads/2021/09/dialogue_and_paradox.pdf.

Kakar, S. (2012). *The inner world: A psychoanalytic study of childhood and society in India* (4th ed.). Oxford University Press.

Kakar, S., & Kakar, K. (2007). *The Indians: Portrait of a people*. Penguin India.

Lyons-Ruth, K. (1999). The two-person unconscious: Intersubjective dialogue, enactive relational representation, and the emergence of new forms of relational organization. *Psychoanalytic Inquiry, 19*(4), 576–617. https://doi.org/10.1080/07351699909534267

Lyons-Ruth, K. (2007). The interface between attachment and intersubjectivity: Perspective from the longitudinal study of disorganized attachment. *Psychoanalytic Inquiry, 26*(4), 595–616. https://doi.org/10.1080/07351690701310656

Lyons-Ruth, K., Bruschweiler-Stern, N., Harrison, A. M., Morgan, A. C., Nahum, J. P., Sander, L., Stern, D. N., & Tronick, E. Z. (1998). Implicit relational knowing: Its role in development and psychoanalytic treatment. *Infant Mental Health Journal, 19*(3), 282–289. https://onlinelibrary.wiley.com/doi/10.1002/(SICI)1097-0355(199823)19:3%3C282::AID-IMHJ3%3E3.0.CO;2-O

Martin, M. (2017). *The dialogical principle in counseling and psychotherapy: An exploration of Martin Buber's 'I and thou'.* JMU Scholarly Commons. https://commons.lib.jmu.edu/edspec201019/113

Morgan, W. J. (2007). Martin Buber: Philosopher of dialogue and of the resolution of conflict. *British Academy Review, 10,* 11–14. www.thebritishacademy.ac.uk/documents/576/04-morgan.pdf.

Orange, D. M. (2009). *Thinking for clinicians: Philosophical resources for contemporary psychoanalysis and the humanistic psychotherapies.* Taylor & Francis.

Orange, D. M., Atwood, G. E., & Stolorow, R. D. (1999). Working intersubjectively: Contextualism in psychoanalytic practice. *Psychoanalytic Psychology, 16*(2), 303–308. https://doi.org/10.1037/0736-9735.16.2.303

Schulz, F. (2004). *Relational Gestalt Therapy: Theoretical foundations and dialogical elements.* https://secureservercdn.net/50.62.174.80/y1a.e81.myftpupload.com/wp-content/uploads/2021/09/RelationalGestaltTherapy.pdf.

Spagnuolo Lobb, M. (2013). Fundamentals and development of gestalt therapy in the contemporary context. In G. Francesetti, M. Gecele, & J. Roubal (Eds.), *Gestalt therapy in clinical practice: From psychopathology to the aesthetics of contact* (pp. 27–57). Istituto di Gestalt HCC Italy.

Stolorow, R. D. (2002). From drive to affectivity: Contextualizing psychological life. *Psychoanalytic Inquiry, 22*(5), 678–685. https://doi.org/10.1080/07351692209349012

Stolorow, R. D. (2008). The contextuality and existentiality of emotional trauma. *Psychoanalytic Dialogues, 18*(1), 113–123. https://doi.org/10.1080/10481880701790133

Stolorow, R. D., Brandchaft, B., & Atwood, G. E. (2014). *Psychoanalytic treatment: An intersubjective approach.* Taylor & Francis/Routledge.

Watson, N. J. (2006). Martin Buber's I and thou: Implications for Christian psychotherapy. *Journal of Psychology and Christianity, 25*(1), 34–43.

Yontef, G., & Fairfield, M. (2008). Gestalt therapy. In K. Jordan (Ed.), *The quick theory reference guide: A resource for expert and novice mental health professionals* (pp. 83–106). Nova Science Publishers.

Yontef, G., & Jacobs, L. (2005). Gestalt therapy. In R. J. Corsini & D. Wedding (Eds.), *Current psychotherapies* (pp. 299–336). Thomson Brooks/Cole.

Yontef, G., & Schulz, F. (2016). Dialogue and experiment. *British Gestalt Journal, 25*(1), 9–21.

Yontef, G. M. (1993). *Awareness, dialogue & process: Essays on gestalt therapy.* Gestalt Journal Press.

Chapter 8

Enduring Relational Themes

Kryptonite

I conduct an annual residential group therapy retreat chiefly for therapists and trainee counselors. This event took place in one of the retreats that I conducted around the time when I was grappling with a life-changing loss. My father, who had been suffering from Alzheimer's for a few years, passed away a week before the retreat. Since I had been grieving for my impending loss for more than ten years, I believed that I could cope with resuming my work after a week. This, of course, was an overvaulting ambition and an error of Macbethian proportion, 'I have no spur to prick the sides of my intent, but only vaulting ambition, which o'erleaps itself, and falls on th'other...' (Shakespeare, 1991, Act 1, scene 7, 25–28). From childhood, my role I believed was of being an emotional support for my mother, so I slipped back into that role easily after my father's death. In fact, as I held my father's face and wept, my mother told me not to cry and disturb him. Her intention was probably to ensure that his face, which was in repose, would not be disturbed (a Hindu custom). However, I remember something shutting down in me. An old message had surfaced, which was to be strong and not cry. After that I went around helping to organize the funeral, attend to the needs of visitors and be a source of succor for my mother while she grieved. Although I spoke to my therapist a few times, this particular theme had slipped my conscious mind and I went to the retreat fully prepared to be the 'ever present and benevolent human being'.

I was disturbed by a few factors during the first day of the retreat, especially, my inability to retain the structure and time frame of the sessions. There were nine participants, I was operating without a co-facilitator, and the session would start early with yoga and meditation, followed by individual pieces and group work interspersed with tea breaks and lunch break. Even though the idea was to wind up by 4:30 p.m., invariably the time got extended by more than an hour on day one. Many of the members felt that they weren't getting enough time with me to resolve what they were working on. I felt inadequate and thought that I was not doing enough, while feeling frustrated with how time seemed to stretch and yet not meet anyone's needs satisfactorily.

DOI: 10.4324/9781003348337-9

I was disturbed enough to sit down and reflect on what was happening. While puzzling about the source of my dilemma, I was struck by how my childhood themes around being 'strong' and 'not being good enough' had resurfaced with a vengeance and had been outside my awareness for more than a week. One of my themes is how to be a 'dharma yogi' (a disciplined practitioner of right action). I used to take my duties and responsibilities to a point of stoic self-neglect. I had worked through many of these themes in my therapy over 20 years; however, the death of my father and my rigid focus on being a good daughter to my grieving widowed mother had led to me slipping back into my old ways of being. As an adult, being a dharma yogi has helped me gain many rewards as a 'superwoman'—partner, mother, daughter, daughter-in-law, friend, sister, student, teacher and therapist. However, the constraints I placed on myself in expressing my feelings and needs were unhelpful as an adult and problematic in my work in the long run.

I first heard the term 'enduring relational themes' (ERTs) during Lynne Jacobs' lecture in 2016 at a residential retreat I was attending at the Pacific Gestalt Institute, California. I was fascinated and thoughtful about how I could use it to understand myself better, and understand my work with individual clients and groups. At the time, I was still trying to find the middle ground between my humanistic existential orientation and my deep allegiance to the psychoanalytic school. I found valuable clinical relevance in classical psychoanalytic conceptualizations postulated by Freud and his followers, and merit in the concept of transference, the object relations school, ego psychology, self-psychology and the intersubjective theory.

In my practice, I had encountered the occurrence of transference and countertransference and appreciated the mindfulness these concepts brought to my work in understanding the therapeutic relationship. Yet I was concerned about its limitations in applying it to a field phenomenological way of working. Jacobs' lecture on ERTs came at an opportune time. I found the notion of ERT easy to grasp, explicit and expansive in its inclusivity of the concept of transference, while remaining true to the dialogic way of working.

ERTs are the leitmotifs we all carry as human beings that are internalized from childhood experiences, which get shaped and reinforced in early relationships and continue to be reformed on an ongoing basis in our encounters with the other. ERTs, as postulated by Jacobs (2017), looks at the recurring patterns in the relational field as an intersubjective process that may have elements of the past; however, it also contains aspects from the here-and-now relationship between the therapist and the client. 'The aspects of the here and now are similar to, or reminiscent of—based on similarity or symbolic significance—the problematic events of the past, even if (hopefully) they are attenuated repetitions' (L. Jacobs, personal communication, 2020). Jacobs (2001) describes how she wanted to make meaning of the themes that emerged in the relationship between the client and the therapist that had either a positive or negative effect on the contacting process. ERTs are described by Jacobs as repetitive, enduring modes of engagement between therapists and clients that can often impose limitations on the range and freedom of contacting that is possible in the therapeutic relationship as well as in the clients' lives. She says that 'from out of this conundrum I have developed over time a practice and a supporting set of ideas around a concept I name "enduring relational themes"' (2017, p. 7).

As mentioned in the earlier chapters of this book, the founders of GT were greatly influenced by their psychoanalytic training and background. Although GT placed primacy on the here-and-now relationship, and the present field in which the client and therapist's experiences take shape, they also emphasized on the early childhood experiences that regulated the present ways of contacting. Laura Perls (1992, as cited in Jacobs, 2017) spoke of the importance of the past and future in how it influences our present:

> [the] emphasis on the Here and Now does not imply, as is so often assumed, that the past and the future are unimportant or nonexistent for Gestalt therapy. On the contrary, the past is ever-present in our total life experience, our memories [...] and particularly in our habits and our hang-ups. [...] The future is present in our preparations and beginnings, in expectation and hope, or dread and despair.
>
> *Perls, p. 149ff., as cited in Staemmler, 2009, p. 198*

One of the most important constructs around how our past that permeates our present life and relationships, especially the therapeutic one, is the concept of transference—Freud's (1912) seminal contribution to the understanding of the therapeutic relationship. I believe it is useful to understand the psychoanalytic concept of transference and countertransference to develop a deeper understanding of ERTs and their value in the practice of GT and GGT.

Transference and Countertransference

Freud hypothesized that past relationships with parental figures could affect the relationship the client had with the therapist. Anna Freud (1954) developed this further by stating that although transference must be meticulously interpreted, the therapist must also be aware that the client and the therapist are two real people of equal status in a real relationship. Branches of the psychoanalytic school, like object relations, self-psychology, and intersubjectivity theorists, further contributed to the etiology and presentation of transference in the analytic relationship, as it moved from a singular intrapsychic process toward a two-person relational and intersubjective model (Parth et al., 2017; Mitchell, 1984; Stolorow, Atwood, & Orange, 2002).

The classical definition of transference was seen as a reenactment of the early childhood Oedipal issues with the father and mother that get transferred onto the therapist in the current therapeutic relationship. Freud (1912) saw transference as a 'template or a central relationship pattern that serves as a prototype or a scheme for shaping subsequent relationships' (Gelso & Hayes, 1998, p. 49). Heimann (1956) proposed that transference, both positive and negative, was an expression of primitive personality content and fantasy that has never before been verbalized by or for the client and its interpretation was pivotal to psychoanalysis (as cited in Parth et al., 2017, p. 188).

Transference can be defined as the client's unconscious allocation of unresolved emotions, sensations, thoughts, beliefs and experiences about significant figures in their early life to the therapist. In the recent developments toward explaining transference by the intersubjective school, this is seen as a co-created reality between the client and therapist that has elements of the past as well as the present. The intersubjective theorists have helped shift the focus from the client's distortions to the therapist's verbal and nonverbal responses, and the meanings this holds for the client. For example, I remember more than a decade ago, a client telling me that they didn't like me not keeping consistent eye contact with them, that my looking out of the French windows intermittently while they talked was rude. I recollect being startled by this feedback because I was not even aware of the impact my action had on their experience of being attended to. For my client, this meant that I was being inattentive, whereas for me it was my way of thinking about what my client was saying and trying to get a sense of how they felt as they narrated their experience. As you can see, my nonverbal response had a specific meaning for my client.

The term 'countertransference' was coined by Freud, and the psychoanalytic view of this is the analyst's unconscious and neurotic 'counter' response to the analysand's transference. The classical definition of countertransference is the therapist's unconscious feelings, thoughts, sensations, beliefs and attitudes that are evoked by the client's transference, and the possible acting out of these by the therapist. However, this classical definition has broadened over time to include all the feelings experienced by the therapist toward the client. Countertransference includes the therapist's repressed, unresolved feelings and attitudes that surface in response to the client's displacement of their own repressed, unresolved experiences. Thus, the definition of countertransference now includes the therapist's unconscious, unresolved emotions and thoughts that are incited by the client's transference, as well as the therapist's conscious, justifiable reactions to actual experiences during therapy. These reactions include those made in response to what the client says and does in therapy, and what they report they are going through outside of therapy (Kernberg, 1987). Heimann (1950) concluded that countertransference is the most valuable tool of assessment into the client's unconscious that the therapist has.

Both transference and countertransference fit well into a Newtonian linear causality view but cannot be easily assimilated into a GT orientation that is grounded on phenomenology and field theory. Moreover, as a concept it is rigid and has a historical inclination toward pathologizing the client while treating the therapist as invincible. White (2008) states that the concepts of transference and countertransference are no longer suitable to us in the practice of contemporary psychotherapy. However, these psychoanalytic concepts related to the therapeutic relationship are vital to the practice of psychotherapy. I believe they are invaluable for the direction they have given us, as well as the opportunity to expand them to suit our work as relational practitioners. Moreover, intersubjective theorists from the psychodynamic school have made considerable contributions to the practice of contemporary psychotherapy by supplementing the concept of transference further. They include Kohut's self-object needs into the here-and-now intersubjective system where emerging experience is seen as co-constructed in the two-person dyad (Goldberg, 1998).

Intersubjective theory is a phenomenological field theory that tries to illuminate the client's transference as not just purely intrapsychic experiences from the past, but rather an interpersonal phenomenon rising from the in-between space of the mutually interacting worlds of the therapist and client. The intersubjective theorists emphasize that psychological phenomena cannot be understood separately from the intersubjective field in which they emerge (Stolorow & Atwood, 1984; Stolorow & Atwood, 1996; Orange, Atwood, & Stolorow, 1999; Stolorow, 1997; Stolorow, Atwood, & Orange, 2002; Stolorow, 2002; Stolorow, 2013). In their conceptualization, 'the patterning of transference is fluid, nonlinear, multidimensional, and dynamically emergent from the self-organizing activity of the patient-analyst system' (Stolorow, 1997, p. 349). This kind of conceptual presentation of the old Freudian concept of transference deconstructs the Cartesian divide and linear causality for a field perspective of the therapist–client relationship. Thus, it moves away from the unachievable classical postulate of an impartial and sterilized container to interpret a client's transference. Also, intersubjectivity is closest to GT in its theoretical assumptions that see the experience of the therapist and client as subjective and equally valid.

Although Gestalt therapists acknowledged the valuable concepts of human personality development that psychoanalytic practitioners brought into the field of psychotherapy practice, they faced difficulty introducing these directly into a Gestalt framework of practice because of the paradigm differences in thinking of both schools. The pioneers of GT tried to detach themselves from their psychoanalytic backgrounds while focusing on the here-and-now relationship between the therapist and client. Although transference was recognized as a phenomenon, classical Gestalt therapists did not see it as necessary to be interpreted or worked through. 'The therapeutic meaning of (transference) is not that it is the same old story, but precisely that it is now differently worked through as a present adventure: the analyst is not the same kind of parent' (*PHG*, 1951, p. 234). However, as contemporary GT moved toward focusing more on the relational component, there has been a renewed and creative reflection on psychoanalytic concepts. Over the years, Gestalt therapists have attempted to assimilate insights from psychoanalytic understandings of transference into the practice of GT. The concepts of transference and countertransference are being looked at with curiosity and theoreticians are creatively exploring the possibilities of its value in GT, to find its meaning within a Gestalt framework (Phillipson, 2002).

According to Jacobs (2017), Gestalt therapists have started to do this because explorations of transference in the psychoanalytic literature have often yielded very rich understandings of clinically relevant relational processes—especially those that occur over time. She adds that transference with all of its baggage, and epistemological and ethical problems, creates trouble when imported into GT; however, the concept of ERTs is an adequate replacement for working with the relationship between our past, our present and our leaning into our future. 'Developing an eye and ear for ERTs, both the hopeful and the dread filled ones, makes the process of finding figures crisper and more salient to the client's therapeutic aims' (p. 16).

Enduring Relational Themes

ERTs is close in its principle with how transference has been postulated by the intersubjective theorists. ERTs are dynamic and triggered within the field co-created by the therapist and client. This kind of approach that is inclusive makes us mindful as therapist/leader to thoughtfully ask the questions 'what am I bringing into this therapeutic field that is activating this response for my client? and what does this client evoke in me of my own themes?', as different from asking the question 'what is the client projecting onto me from her unresolved childhood?' For example, when a member in the group experiences me as distant to her expression of anger—it may be triggering for her past experiences of coldness/withdrawal of a significant other and it is also a here-and-now experience, because I can on rare occasions slip into my ERT of anxiety and withdrawal when I perceive rage in the other.

In my individual practice as well as my work with groups, I have often been aware of how our respective ERTs surface in the intersubjective field between me and my clients. In the vignette, 'Kryptonite', my theme about my not being 'good enough' surfaced, just as some members felt I was not doing enough to be available to meet their needs, which were their themes with their early caregivers. The emergence of ERTs is inevitable and the resulting rupture is often unavoidable. However, the awareness of it accompanied with a dialogic attitude can facilitate repair of the disruption in the contacting process. This informs our practice to be focused toward creating new ERTs that are more flexible and supportive of the client's relational needs. Before illustrating an example of ERT and how it is addressed in GGT, it is useful to gain a thorough understanding of the concept of ERT, and how it differs from the classical conceptualization of transference and countertransference.

Enduring

The word 'enduring' is quite self-explanatory as it means something that persists over time and is long established as opposed to something that is transient and fleeting. Jacobs (2017) uses the term 'enduring' because these are repetitive, steady over time and many are distinctive styles of self-protection. In an early relational field with significant figures, the child creatively adjusts to the demands of the environment that becomes a template for future interactions. These adjustments are dynamic yet they are also repetitive and pervasive. The painful outcomes that stem from these recurrent themes are what often makes clients seek therapy, for example, the tenacious feelings of inadequacy, recurrent loss of intimate relationships or persistent difficulties at work. However, ERTs are not inert residues of the unfinished past; rather, they are internalized in the past, continue to get strengthened or weakened through ongoing life experiences, and they enable our journey into the future. We move onward hopefully in our life's journey, in search of healing relationships and closure for our woundedness, and this is an incremental process of movement into our next adjacent possible.

Relational

The word 'relational' has two different references, according to Jacobs. The first reference is to the fact that our ERTs grow and are sustained or tested within a relationship. If we have had repetitive experiences in childhood of our feelings invalidated, then they get solidified into certain ways of being in relationships. For example, a young boy who grew up in an environment where the female figures were harsh and ridiculing, now as an adult member of a group consisting of mostly female figures may feel that they are harsh each time they express their anger toward men. As a group leader, when we explore or give a language to these feelings, we consistently behave differently in a way that challenges these experiences, and when other group members respond to this with honesty, without trying to be reassuring or defensive, then a new ERT around safety with female figures can develop. This is similar to what Lyons-Ruth (1998) refers to as relational knowing. Often therapy offers a space for experiences that are reparative of the past woundedness and support the development of new ways of being in a relationship. This process helps create a flexibility in stuck Gestalts and what Fairbairn (1958) has called 'closed systems', while referring to the internal world of the client that has become obdurate due to repetitive experience of trauma (as cited in Reubens, 1984). Harrow (2020) says that this closed system involves perpetuation of relationships between aspects of the self and respective internal objects, as well as between one another. I believe therapy offers restorative experiences that open up the closed systems, which can lead to a pliability in assimilating new experiences and moving forward in creative ways. This does not imply that earlier ERTs vanish, but over time, as newer ERTs develop, the more rigid ones tend to recede in importance unless the client undergoes a particularly stressful situation (Jacobs, 2017).

The second reference for 'relational' is that all ERTs suggest the impact of the 'other'. I agree with Jacobs (2017) that this second reference is critical in the therapy process. All of us have familiar relational modes of dealing with stress, anxiety, loneliness, fears of rejection and hopes of acceptance. Clients often seek therapy to get closure for unfinished experiences from the past where they have experienced deprivation. They may repeat the creative adjustments from their early relationships hoping for a new relational experience. Therapists are also prone to responding from their own ERTs. The therapist's job is to understand these themes of self and client dialogically so that new creative ways of relating with the other can be experimented with. As human beings, we hope for disconfirmation of our beliefs that we will be hurt or rejected if we express our true selves, yet we despair that our needs will be met. By responding to a client relationally, there is a possibility in therapy to disconfirm the client's dread and confirm the hope. Since ERTs indicate the presence of the 'other', when a visible and figural ERT occurs in a therapy session, as the therapist it behooves us to explore the role we played in the emergence of this theme. In fact, when a client is reacting to the therapist with one of their more anguished ERTs, the therapist's exploration and acknowledgment of their participation in the evocation of that theme is often one of the most powerful antidotes through which a new theme that counters the dread-filled theme can develop (Jacobs, 2017).

Theme

The word 'theme', as it suggests, captures the repetitive embodied, symbolic ways of relating, responding and reacting in our worlds, like a musical score. It's a combination of our emotional, cognitive and behavioral functions that play out in the ways we connect with ourselves, the other and the world in a recurrent manner. Jacobs (2017) says that these emotional and action patterns carry symbols and imagery that can be expressed through language; when the therapist and client mutually find the right words, images, and figures it can become a relational event of meaning making in itself. I want to share with you here an example from my work that I think can explain this process further. I often use expressive art in both individual and group settings, and I find the rosebush activity quite useful in developing an awareness of the client's relational themes. The rosebush (Allan, 1988; Birch & Carmichael, 2009) is a Jungian guided imagery activity that is primarily used to work with children to explore their inner world. I use this at times in groups to facilitate awareness and engage in a dialogue with each member. Often, the drawing of the self as a rose is unique to each individual member and I have seen inimitable responses to this prompt. For some, the symbol is accompanied with the presence of other roses along with the self, trees, bushes, houses, churches, temples and other elements both man-made and natural. Some of the members experience threat and isolation when working with the metaphor. Some narrate experiences of growing wild in the jungle, dependent on the vagaries of nature to nurture them, stagnant as the seasons change, and a fear of being annihilated. Some members feel a sense of protection with their thorns, a connection to nature, safety and belongingness as they feel nurtured by their deep roots as well as the presence of a gardener. Some find the thorns unwanted or disturbing, fearing it will hurt them or others and further add to their feelings of isolation. Some members have mixed experiences of declining, withering as well as of renewal and recovery. As a leader, I try to find the individual meaning making for each member and the emergent themes from their imagery.

I have found the rosebush yields specific individual responses as well as universal themes around experiences of the self in relation to one's family, and how this surfaces in group relationships now. Some have had experiences of threat, sibling rivalry and lack of safety in the extended family system. Others have had experiences of connectedness, warmth and cohesiveness with neighborhood groups even if within the family there was isolation. One participant who expressed wanting to grow wild amid deep woods, felt acutely the fear of isolation as well as the fear of intimacy. He found it difficult to navigate his boundaries within the group, which was his experience in his intimate and work relationships outside the group as well. When he became aware of this through the metaphor of a rosebush, it had a significant impact on how he tested his relationships and developed connections with the group members. The imagery of the rosebush is quite a useful symbolic activity for individual clients as well as members of GGT. I have found that in a group setting, this activity helps us find a language to express the emergent themes and build awareness into how these unique themes regulate our perceptual experiences in a relationship, moment to moment.

How obdurate ERTs can be depends on the degree, repetitiveness and intensity of trauma that we may have gone through in our childhood and the fixed Gestalts varies from individual to individual in its rigid nature depending on the force of trauma. These ERTs are rigid because they are the internal organizations that influence how we perceive our self, the other and the world. We may have internal beliefs about the self, like 'I am irreparably flawed/stupid/helpless'. Or we may have themes about how we perceive others, like a belief that 'People are not safe. Others are out to get me. No one will care for me'. Then there are refrains that reflect how we experience the world, like 'The world is dangerous and merciless. I must keep my guard up and protect myself from the world at all times'. These are all examples of fixed, emotionally laden beliefs that become centerpieces of the therapeutic process, including how we experience the therapeutic relationship (Jacobs, 2017).

Jacobs (2017) goes on to add that all ERTs are not negative beliefs and expectations. I believe this to be true. I grew up in a unique matrilineal society in the south of India during the 1970s, with patriarchal nuances, and during this time women could exercise a fair amount of independence, especially in the areas of property inheritance, education and pursuit of a career. So, within the larger context of the patriarchal society that marks Indian culture generally, where women are encouraged to be the epitome of virtuous self-sacrifice, I personally developed a sense of assurance in my pursuit of knowledge. This gives me a profound sense of confidence and pride in the way I walk through life with a sense of agency that I can will things to happen. Along with this I have my fair share of ERTs around being pridefully independent, 'a misfit' and the accompanied loneliness of not belonging to the larger cultural community.

The brutally challenging ERTs are the ones that limit and truncate our freedom, and they represent self-preservation and survival tactics that develop in a barren, punishing or depriving environment. For example, in Emily Brontë's (1847/1992) *Wuthering Heights*, the male protagonist, Heathcliff, is an orphan child who is adopted and treated with care by Mr. Earnshaw. Earnshaw dies when Heathcliff is a young adolescent, and the oldest son, Hindley, is cuttingly abusive to young Heathcliff. Heathcliff grows up to become an arrogant, sensitive, moody and cruel man. Brontë compares Heathcliff, who has an impoverished and punitive childhood, to the gaunt thorns stunted by the repetitive cruelty of stormy winds and nature. In such an arid and punishing field there is a dearth of opportunity for the child to develop emotional, cognitive and active skills. Moreover, the capacity to self-regulate and the learned ability of how to be in relationships, or what Lyons-Ruth calls 'relational knowing', is overwhelmingly challenged. The ability to perceive the self as lovable, the other as fairly loving, the world as a relatively safe place, and the ability to relate with the other gets compromised. The capacity to be creative in contacting the other for one's relational needs is fragmented. These become fixed Gestalts that limit the individual's dexterity at deriving alternative meanings from the behaviors of others.

This is what Jacobs (2017) calls a totalistic environment from which escape is almost futile, if not impossible, and where ERTs are rigidly cemented. For example, a child may have learned to be aggressive or withdrawing when they found the environment threatening or punishing. This was a creative adjustment when the child first engaged in this behavior. In a therapeutic situation, the client may respond to the therapist with aggression or withdrawal when they experience a threat that the therapist may say and do something overpowering or hurtful. This is further exacerbated by not having the semantic knowledge of how to express the dread of being wounded, or even the dread of wounding the other and being abandoned for it. For example, when I say to my client, 'I wonder what you fear the most, the fear of being hurt by me, or terror of being abandoned if you hurt me?', this opens up opportunities to give a language to the felt anxieties of the client. An understanding of ERTs helps the therapist develop sensitivity toward the client's themes and explore and offer a language to make sense of these themes, while responding in a manner that is contrary to past experiences. This then provides an alternative relational experience that enables and supports a forward movement in healing from past trauma.

I believe that ERT as a singular phrase is inclusive of the relational dynamics between the therapist and the client that supports a deeper understanding of the psychotherapeutic relationship. The basic premise that both the therapist and the client have ERTs that can be triggered in a relational field somehow reduces the shame the client may otherwise feel in an approach that sees transference as a projection of the client's unresolved past onto the therapist. Although shame as an experience is unavoidable, I think as therapists it is important for us to be attuned to how it can be easily triggered and the role we may play in its occurrence. As a therapist, an effective way to lower the chances of this kind of damage is by developing a familiarity with our own ERTs, practicing self-awareness and engaging in personal therapy that helps develop creative, supple and adaptive ways of relating with the self, the other and the world. This enhances the therapist's ability to be sensitive to the client's ERTs. Awareness and approximate resolution of one's own ERTs facilitates openness toward exploring the unique ERTs that each client can bring, and nurturing a genuine curiosity toward making meaning of what the client is trying to verbally or nonverbally communicate.

The group as a therapeutic setting widens the scope of alternative relational experiences because there are other members whose presence reduces the perceived power of the therapist. The other members can often provide different perspectives and feedback that brings a universality to one's experiences, challenges fixed Gestalts and opens up the horizon for developing new ways of being and relating.

ERTs in a Group Setting

With my work, in general and with this group retreat in particular (Kryptonite), I am what Jung (1966) called the Mother Archetype. Tower (1956) says that this a relevant archetype to therapy because, like the prototypical mother–child relationship, therapy involves repeated and intimate contact between two persons through conscious and unconscious channels of communication. He says that therapy becomes an opportunity for therapists to play the maternal role of creating and nourishing new psychic life, and that therapists who unconsciously hold the belief that they are and should be benevolent and self-giving and that clients should be able to use their therapists to obtain whatever they need, are especially vulnerable to acting out the Mother

Archetype. I slipped into this theme, my maternal side, with a fairly conscious belief that I should be giving and nourishing. This part of me that is nurturing is usually helpful for me as a therapist. It keeps me empathetic toward my clients. However, it can also generate subjective distress and interpersonal conflict, especially when it is practiced without consciously setting limits and regulating boundaries. The closest I can come to explaining this conundrum is through a Malayalam proverb my grandmother would often use when I was in her care, *'adhikamayal amritham visham'* (in excess even elixir is poison). As I continued to give more to compensate for some of the participants' ERTs of the mother not giving enough and being unavailable, I started stretching my limits. As a theme this continued to emerge in the individual pieces of work a few of them did—mothers or fathers who weren't emotionally and physically available, who were distant, neglectful and highly critical. My attempts to wind up on time or close a piece of work that the member then experienced as a lack of resolution was evocative of a mother who could not fulfill their needs. The members' responses in turn touched my theme of not 'being good enough' and 'strong enough', and the dread that whatever I do, I cannot satisfy the 'other'.

I realized how my ERTs interacted with some of the participants' ERTs, creating a fertile field for therapeutic misattunement, shame, as well as humbling self-awareness for me. It was the first group that I conducted that ended on a disturbingly open note, where we carried back a sense of shame and lack of closure from the retreat. Fortunately for us, we were able to address these residual feelings in an ongoing process group that they were part of, where these concerns were talked about and ruptures repaired over time. I had sufficient support from my supervisor to process my shame about slipping into my ERTs, not being a perfect therapist, and between us we held my shame with compassionate humor. I took responsibility for my own difficulty in going outside the structure on day one, which was reminiscent of my confluence with my mother. My attempts to meet their needs at the cost of not being attuned to my needs was unhelpful to us. The participants had a willingness and humor to look into what they wanted from me and how they felt disappointed when I wouldn't meet all their needs, and I was able to hold their grief about not having a good enough 'mother'.

The way I moved between giving too much out of overvaulting ambition and then moving away, dreading depletion, were redolent of my ERTs surrounding how I cope with external and internal demands. I think what was helpful was also my supportive ERTs about how relationships can be repaired—an intrinsic belief that with acceptance and humor, amends are a possibility, that once we rest, recuperate and reflect, we can come back with a renewed energy for repairing ruptures.

Each one of us as a human being, by virtue of our humanity, has unresolved issues that can trigger personal ERTs. As therapists, we are not immune to our ERTs, despite therapy and supervision. ERTs can still be activated when a significant event occurs and it touches our lives deeply. When this is outside the awareness of the therapist and not attended to with immediacy, it can negatively impact the process of therapy. Qualities that help minimize the acting out of ERTs include the therapist's level of self-integration and acceptance, accompanied with the ability to recognize, tolerate and manage shame, and the ability to formulate an understanding and meaning making of the transpired event. This is arduous work with individuals, and more so with groups, because it involves the ability to swim in the painful prevailing tides of many narratives with each person's unique ERTs coming together. The willingness to share another's suffering when the human impulse is to escape pain, can be quite challenging. What supports group leaders in this process is having a scaffolding from one's supervisor and therapist when needed, and sustaining presence and dialogue with the members of the group. It is accepting that as humans we make errors, and it is our self-awareness and openness to access supportive relationships that help us make amends.

References

Allan, J. A. B. (1988). *Inscapes of the child's world: Jungian counseling in schools and clinics*. Spring Publications.

Birch, J., & Carmichael, K. D. (2009). Using drawings in play therapy: A Jungian approach. *The Alabama Counseling Association Journal, 34*(2), 2–7.

Brontë, E. (1847/1992). *Wuthering Heights*. Knopf Doubleday.

Fairbairn, W. R. D. (1958). On the nature and aims of psycho-analytical treatment. *International Journal of Psychoanalysis, 39*, 374–385.

Freud, A. (1954). The widening scope of indications for psychoanalysis discussion. *Journal of the American Psychoanalytic Association, 2*(4), 607–620. https://doi.org/10.1177/000306515400200404

Freud, S. (1912). The dynamics of transference. In J. Strachey (Trans.), *The standard edition of the complete psychological works of Sigmund Freud* (Vol. 12, pp. 99–108). Hogarth Press.

Gelso, C. J., & Hayes, J. A. (1998). *The psychotherapy relationship: Theory, research, and practice*. John Wiley & Sons.

Goldberg, A. (1998). Self psychology since Kohut. *Psychoanalytic Quarterly, 67*(2), 240–255. https://doi.org/10.1080/21674086.1998.11927558

Harrow, J. A. (2020). Towards a theory of the self: Fairbairn and beyond. In F. Pereira & D. E. Scharff (Eds.), *Fairbairn and relational theory* (pp. 183–196). Routledge.

Heimann, P. (1950). On counter-transference. *International Journal of Psychoanalysis, 31*, 81–84.

Heimann, P. (1956). Dynamics of transference interpretation. *International Journal of Psychoanalysis, 37*, 303–310.

Jacobs, L. (2001). Pathways to a relational worldview. In M. R. Goldfried (Ed.), *How therapists change: Personal and professional reflections* (pp. 271–288). American Psychological Association.

Jacobs, L. (2017). Hopes, fears, and enduring relational themes. *British Gestalt Journal, 26*(1), 7–16.

Jung, C. G. (1966). *The archetypes and the collective unconscious* (Vol. 9). Princeton University Press.

Kernberg, O. F. (1987). An ego psychology-object relations theory approach to the transference. *Psychoanalytic Quarterly, 56*(1), 197–221. https://doi.org/10.1080/21674086.1987.11927172

Lyons-Ruth, K., Bruschweiler-Stern, N., Harrison, A. M., Morgan, A. C., Nahum, J. P., Sander, L., Stern, D. N., & Tronick, E. Z. (1998). Implicit relational knowing: Its role in development and psychoanalytic treatment. *Infant Mental Health Journal, 19*(3), 282–289. https://onlinelibrary.wiley.com/doi/abs/10.1002/%28SICI%291097-0355%28199823%2919%3A3%3C282%3A%3AAID-IMHJ3%3E3.0.CO%3B2-O

Mitchell, S. A. (1984). Object relations theories and the developmental tilt. *Contemporary Psychoanalysis, 20*(4), 473–499. https://doi.org/10.1080/00107530.1984.10745749

Orange, D. M., Atwood, G. E., & Stolorow, R. D. (1999). *Working intersubjectively: Contextualism in psychoanalytic practice*. Analytic Press.

Parth, K., Datz, F., Seidman, C., & Löffler-Stastka, H. (2017). Transference and countertransference: A review. *Bulletin of the Menninger Clinic, 81*(2), 167–211. https://doi.org/10.1521/bumc.2017.81.2.167

Perls, F. S., Goodman, P., & Hefferline, R. F. (1951). *Gestalt therapy: Excitement and growth in the human personality*. Dell.

Perls, L. (1992). *Living at the boundary: The collected works of Laura Perls*. (J. Wysong, Ed.). Gestalt Journal Press.

Philippson, P. (2002). A gestalt therapy approach to transference. *British Gestalt Journal, 11*(1), 16–20.

Rubens, R. L. (1984). The meaning of structure in Fairbairn. *International Review of Psycho-Analysis, 11*(4), 429–440.

Shakespeare, W. (1964). Macbeth. In *The complete works of William Shakespeare: Quatercentenary edition* (pp. 999–1027). The English Language Book Society and Collins.

Staemmler, F.-M. (2009). *Aggression, time, and understanding: Contributions to the evolution of gestalt therapy*. Gestalt Press/Routledge.

Stolorow, R. D. (1997). Dynamic, dyadic, intersubjective systems: An evolving paradigm for psychoanalysis. *Psychoanalytic Psychology, 14*(3), 337–346. https://doi.org/10.1037/h0079729

Stolorow, R. D. (2002). Impasse, affectivity, and intersubjective systems. *Psychoanalytic Review, 89*(3), 329–337. https://doi.org/10.1521/prev.89.3.329.22075

Stolorow, R. D. (2013). Intersubjective-systems theory: A phenomenological-contextualist psychoanalytic perspective. *Psychoanalytic Dialogues, 23*(4), 383–389. https://doi.org/10.1080/10481885.2013.810486

Stolorow, R. D., & Atwood, G. E. (1984). Psychoanalytic phenomenology: Toward a science of human experience. *Psychoanalytic Inquiry, 4*(1), 87–105. https://doi.org/10.1080/07351698409533532

Stolorow, R. D., & Atwood, G. E. (1996). The intersubjective perspective. *Psychoanalytic Review, 83*(2), 181–194.

Stolorow, R., Atwood, G., & Orange, D. (2002). *Worlds of experience: Interweaving philosophical and clinical dimensions in psychoanalysis*. Basic Books.

Tower, L. E. (1956). Countertransference. *Journal of the American Psychoanalytic Association, 4*(2), 224–255. https://doi.org/10.1177/000306515600400202

White, C. (2008). *Beyond transference: Towards a psychotherapy for the 21st century.* ResearchGate.   www.researchgate.net/profile/Colin-White/publication/338967039_ Beyond_transference_Towards_a_psychotherapy_for_the_21st_century/links/ 5e3567e6a6fdccd9657c760d/Beyond-transference-Towards-a-psychotherapy-for- the-21st-century.pdf.

Chapter 9

Experimentation

Bataka

I remember my personal experience as a participant of a therapy group more than two decades ago. It was a five-day residential retreat with my fellow trainees and the group leader, who had been invited to India to conduct group therapy for our batch. The leader was new to us; however, we (the participants) had been in a process-oriented training group for around two years, knew each other's stories, had worked on some of our issues with different therapists, and we shared a fair level of comfort and camaraderie with each other. We all had the opportunity to volunteer to do individual pieces of work with the leader and I recollect all of us being enthusiastic about doing our personal work. There was a combination of techniques used like psychodrama, empty chair, and bataka bat to give expression to experiences and trapped emotions. In the personal work I did, the leader suggested I use the bataka bat to express my anger toward a parental figure. Anger for me was then, and is to some extent now, a difficult emotion to express—partially because of my temperament and probably due to my early role models, gender conditioning and cultural background. So, using the bataka bat to hit a bolster was an uncomfortable experience for me. My peers were very supportive, the group leader was encouraging and helpful, but I still struggled to really get into the act. My memory of doing this piece of work is of an awkward, stiff young woman not wanting to disappoint my peers and leader while not wanting to disrespect my parents—a conundrum.

As I was recollecting this incident for this book, I also wondered if it was fear, loneliness and grief I needed to express? And anger toward myself! However, I believe that the work with the leader and group support did help me overcome some social inhibitions and started me on a journey of being more expressive in groups. This vignette is an example of how experimentation was practiced a few decades ago, probably when group therapy as a modality arrived in India in the 1980s and started getting famous in 1990s. At that time, I think encounter groups and techniques from GT were just gaining popularity in some of the training programs in India and we were

DOI: 10.4324/9781003348337-10

attracting faculty from the Western countries to come and train us in working with groups using GT techniques.

Experimentation in GT

The Oxford dictionary defines experiment as 'a scientific procedure undertaken to make a discovery, test a hypothesis, or demonstrate a known fact'. The word 'experiment' is derived from the Latin word *experiri*, which means 'to try', and it is an act taken on to discover some unknown principle or effect. It has been part of GT from the time of its origins in the 1950s with the experimental techniques developed by *PHG* (1951), which brought a fresh zeal into the understanding of human personality. *PHG* was envisioned to support therapists to go beyond their divisive approach toward assessment and treatment, and assimilate new perspectives to the understanding of psychological distress and intervention. It was intended to provide psychotherapists with the tools to support the field phenomenological approach by offering expressive activities for awareness, contact, personal development and integration.

   PHG (1951) says that the very act of therapeutic interview is an experiment. For example, when I ask my client, 'how are you feeling as you tell me this painful story at this moment?' or say, 'I notice that your breathing looks difficult as you share your experiences with me, I wonder what is happening to you now?', these questions are an experiment that is geared toward facilitating the development of awareness. The intention of an experiment in GT is to invite the client to experience 'the actual living through an event' (*PHG*, 1951, p. 15) without just merely talking about it. The way we feel and perceive experiences has a profound impact on how we respond, and our living through these experiences brings awareness into our self, and we are influenced by and we influence our environment. The client's way of being has a subjective impact on me just as the client is impacted by me, for example, when I respond to my client with how I am impacted, 'as I hear your story, I feel pain, I am sorry this happened to you'. The concept of scientific objectivity in experimentation is not present here because I am part of the experiment.

   As a therapist, I introduce an experiment with an invitation, 'would you like to try this out and see what happens?' to facilitate awareness through doing rather than speaking about something. As Roubal (2009) says, an experiment in GT is about doing and direct experience rather than thinking about and description. Being able to relive emotions and affective states and having another human being who will empathize and support the meaning making of these experiences is an important part of GT. Experiments act as doors to build awareness into the internal world of ERTs and help make them figural, and change is often a by-product of this process. Hence, it's imperative that therapists have a good understanding and working knowledge of how experiments and a dialogic attitude work in tandem.

Potential for Application

Polster (2005) distinguishes awareness, contact and experiment as the three fundamental therapeutic instruments of GT (as cited in Roubal, 2019). I believe experiments are the creative tools by which we explore the client's phenomenal field and meet our client in the therapeutic relationship. I use the word 'creative' deliberately because experimental attitude is part of the ongoing dialogue that rises organically to explore what is emerging in the therapy process. I agree with Gestalt practitioners that the experiments are not canned techniques that the therapist takes down from the clinician's shelf to prescribe like medication to reduce symptoms (Brownell, 2010; Greenberg & Kahan, 1978; Fogarty et al., 2016; Yontef & Jacobs, 2005; Yontef & Schulz, 2016). To summarize Hycner (1985), techniques emerge from the relationship between therapist and client. He says that the 'between' is parallel to the Gestalt idea that the 'whole', which is the dialogic realm, is greater than the sum of its 'parts', which is the therapist and client in this context. I agree with him that without a dialogic attitude, experimentation can turn into an activity that hangs awkwardly in the air without really achieving the potential it has to bring alive clients' experiences in the moment.

To quote Mann (2010),

> An experiment is a useful figural exercise in GT that will fall into the ground of the therapeutic relationship. For instance, an experiment that facilitates an expression of anger at an authority figure can lead to a reconfiguration of the client's field in relation to his expressing strong emotion. Such a change occurs in the ground as new embedded awareness sediments down, replacing past creative adjustments.
>
> *p. 134*

I believe the ability and process of the client to express anger at an authority figure facilitates awareness and change. However, this can happen only in a safe relationship with the therapist who is committed to a dialogue with the client.

Experiments have great potential to bring awareness to the client as well as the therapist about how past feelings, bodily sensations, thoughts and enculturation can continue to influence the present experience. For example, in 'Bataka', my reluctance to express anger was greatly influenced by my past and this discomfort was something I was aware of in the present, but at that time I did not possess a language to communicate my discomfort. That our past influences both our present and future is agreed upon across most psychotherapy schools. *PHG* (1951) says that in the last years of his life, Freud stated that no practice could be called psychoanalysis that did not facilitate the recovery of the infantile memory. According to *PHG*, from a GT perspective, what Freud meant was that 'a large part of the unaware self is still acting out the unfinished situations' (p. 291).

In the traditional psychoanalytic approach, the therapist tried creating a neutral therapeutic environment, encouraging free association and transference interpretation to support recovery of infantile memory. Although behaviorism and cognitive psychology saw behaviors and cognitions as having been shaped in childhood, it considered present behavior and cognitive functions as the area for modifications. Both schools followed the Cartesian mind–body divide, where either the psyche or observable actions or functions of the mind were seen as the issue to work on in therapy. The person was not seen as a whole that is inclusive of mind, body, emotions, sensations and belief systems in relation to the sociocultural context (inclusive of that of the therapist), which impacts and is impacted by them.

GT believes that the mind, behavior, body and environment cannot be divided into separate entities and scientifically studied or modified by an observer since they are essentially interlinked. In fact, the observer and the observed influence each other, and I agree with *PHG* (1951) that we blandly commit what to the experimentalist is the most unpardonable of sins by including the experimenter in the experiment. I think dialogue is a prerequisite to understanding this intersubjective phenomenon. In a dialogic experimental approach, the therapist is attuned to the emotionally laden painful ERTs of the client, those especially triggered by the therapist, while using experiments in a safe situation to make clients' primeval experiences salient in the here and now. As therapists, we may have observed that at times repetitive narrations of an old story or ongoing recollections by a client can tend to be lacking in life, 'verbal reminiscing tends to be dry and lifeless, for the past consists of unchangeable particulars. It becomes alive only when it is related to present needs that have some possibility of change' (*PHG*, 1951, p. 306).

RGT has integrated the robust psychoanalytic understanding of early relational experiences of the client, GT's field phenomenological approach, dialogue and creative experimentation to support the client's awareness and growth process. Experiments can give rise to new understanding; illuminate internal boundaries of thinking, feeling and sensations; and develop the potential to imaginatively relate with the world. Yontef and Schulz (2016) say that the suggestion of an experiment is itself an experiment in terms of how the client responds—for example, the ability to say 'no' to a suggestion may develop the client's capacity to resist authority figures. They say that exploring the hesitation of a client to participate is much more important than the performance of an experiment because exploration itself creates awareness.

I think this is an important idea to keep in mind, especially so in the Indian cultural context. As therapists, if we have internalized hierarchy, which is outside our conscious awareness, then we may be susceptible to taking offense when the client refuses to participate in an experiment. Rather than exploring the client's hesitation to engage in an experiment (which can have complex cultural aspects), we may fall prey to labeling the client 'resistant'. I think that the word 'resistant' has an implication that the client is obstinately trying to avoid the therapist's attempts to do what is helpful for him. This may not be necessarily true, because as human beings we are rarely aware of how we adapted to our early environment, how we still use these adaptations to respond to our present, and its influences on our relationships and future. In addition, I believe as humans we are ill-equipped to try out new ways of relating to our world, because we often lack the procedural knowledge of doing so. Experiments illuminate the fixed Gestalts that are outside our awareness, and a client's hesitation or compliance to do an experiment may have been the creative adjustment they made as a child in a challenging environment. By carefully creating experiments with the client, the adaptations of early childhood can be explored and lived experientially in the here and now, and I agree with Mann (2010) that it can free up space for the formation of a new experience.

An experiment might be dramatic or liberating; however, 'its goal is greater awareness, not a directed change in the client's behaviour and the exploration aims for self-recognition and self-acceptance, and not self-denial, self-rejection, or self-hate' (Yontef & Fuhr, 2005, p. 83). Experiments emerge from the moment to enhance the client's awareness of their present struggles and how this might be shaped by their past experiences. Gestalt therapists give primacy to the therapeutic relationship as a decisive factor in healing. The therapist creates a safe space, through the 'I-Thou' mode of meeting, for developing awareness into the fixed Gestalts of the client. I believe this evolving awareness into rigid patterns of relating, opens the door for the adjacent possibilities for the client. To facilitate this process, experimentation is used for developing mindfulness into one's relationship with self, others and the world at large.

Having shared a brief history, rationale and potential of experimentation in GT, I think it's important for me to share with my readers my ambivalence about writing this chapter and the reasons for it. In India, GT techniques are taught as a prescriptive tool in the course curriculum of psychotherapy approaches, unfortunately turning it into a misrepresentation of Gestalt experimental approach. Students of psychology frequently use empty chair in their internship period for 'forgiveness' work with clients who have unfinished anger toward parents, and twin chair for any 'top dog' and 'underdog' conflicts, with the aim of letting go of anger, to resolve internal dilemmas and silence the internal critical voice. Twin chair and empty chair are as much a part of the Indian psychology student's common vocabulary and practice as the analytic concepts of free association and transference. It's a matter of concern for me that the rich potential of GT gets missed in this kind of theoretical truncation. I agree with Laura Perls (1992) that GT gets reduced to a mere technicality and it gets combined with other forms of therapy that are available to us in our armamentarium. To summarize her, we receive sensitivity training and Gestalt, body awareness and Gestalt, transactional analysis and Gestalt, and something or other and Gestalt ad infinitum.

Whether novice or seasoned practitioners, most of us genuinely wish to help our clients and we may feel helpless or inadequate when we are not able to, which can prompt us to use experiments to relieve the clients' distress. Yontef and Schulz (2016) say that when the concept of experiment is introduced, especially to trainee therapists, they get excited by its concrete applicational value because the broader concepts of phenomenology, existentialism, and dialogic method might at times seem vague or lacking in specificity in application. 'The pressures on therapists to find solutions, to help or to relieve painful symptomatology are not insignificant, and they can become powerful motivations to move the therapy in a particular direction rather than to work alongside the client' (p. 18).

Risks of Experimentation

During the sixties and seventies, when GT was becoming popular, the innovative experiments of Perls like empty chair and exaggerations became frozen into dangerous procedures as a cure and became larger than the relational factors (Melnick, 1980; Melnick & Nevis, 1997; Yontef, 1993). The Third Force therapies favored active techniques, often modeled on and advocating confrontational modes of relating that were mostly theatrical, abrasive and/or organized around cathartic experiments (Yontef, 2007; Yontef & Schulz, 2016). These techniques encouraged intense emotional expressions that led to dramatic outcomes. Clients screamed, confronted each other in groups, did exaggerated bodywork, used the bataka encounter bat for emotional release and they dialogued with empty chairs. We can see how this trickled down to India by the eighties and still continues to be practiced here.

The therapeutic interventions as they were practiced in traditional GT, included active and authentic involvement of the therapist, with a focus on contemporaneity and concerted attention to the awareness process with body, sensation, affect and movement, as opposed to neutrally interpreting the unconscious (Yontef & Schulz, 2016). However, these active techniques frequently generated shame and additional damage to the self-esteem of the participants, especially the psychologically vulnerable population. For example, some of these GT methods were paradoxical in terms of emphasizing individuality and assertion, but used techniques that encouraged conformity. Similarly, some theories of therapeutic relationships encouraged client self-esteem while using experiments that were shaming (Jacobs, 1989; Yontef, 1993). Other schools of psychotherapy incorporated techniques like awareness exercises, empty chair and enactments into their practice, often taking it out of the GT framework and using it for behavioral change. Thus, experimentation became geared toward behavior modification, instead of facilitating phenomenological awareness. Over time, classical GT came to be known for its transformative techniques and unfortunately, the essence of its theory and practice receded in value. From the viewpoint of other psychotherapeutic approaches, GT still has the unfortunate reputation of an approach that is based on experiments. RGT moved away significantly from these classical GT techniques because of the risks involved in this methodology and renewed its focus on the therapeutic relationship rather than dramatic experiments.

These concerns around the reduction of Gestalt experiments for behavior modification, and apprehension that the experiments given here would be used without creating a safe therapeutic relationship have contributed to my ambivalence. However, I do see a paradox here. I fear that if I write this chapter, then it has the potential to be misused, and if I avoid writing this chapter, it would mean that the existing knowledge in India about GT and its practice would continue to be maintained, with its limitations. In addition, in the last few decades of my career as a teacher of psychology in Bangalore, India, I have come across many promising students who are curious and creative, have a quest for knowledge and are quite dedicated to their personal and professional development. So, I hope this chapter supports their quest and is not taken out of the context of this book and I trust that the 'part' is used while being attentive to the 'whole'. I hope our work is informed by mindfulness that the experiments are embedded in the I-Thou relationship intended toward awareness and not behavioral change.

I hope that a procedural knowledge of the ethical and professional qualities needed to do experimentation with a relational mindset will help practitioners be better equipped in practicing GT in its true spirit. To summarize Mann (2010), the boundaries of creative experimentation are agreed in the therapeutic relationship between client and therapist and are shaped by existing field conditions including moral and ethical boundaries. There are some important ethical, moral and relational considerations for the therapist to be mindful of before suggesting an experiment.

Attitude of Therapist

As has been discussed extensively in chapter 4, the self of the therapist is a crucial component in therapeutic practice and outcome of therapy. Therapist attitude, beliefs, values and level of self-awareness play a significant role in how the therapeutic dyad engages in experimentation. The therapist must develop the ability to establish contact with self as well as the client, and this ability to invest in the contacting process supports the creation of a safe emergency for the therapeutic encounter. Safe because the space needs to be well contained, structured and inclusive, yet the experiment is an emergency because it entails doing something that can be scary as it involves going into an unknown territory.

Contact and Safe Emergency

Buber's dialogic existentialism, as elaborated in chapter 7 of this book, is an explicit form of contact that is appropriate for therapists who work relationally. When we incorporate experimentations into the relational qualities of inclusion, presence and dialogue, then there is an obvious implication that the therapist contacts the client where they are in their reality, journeys with the client's experience and does not try to change the client. Yontef (1993) elaborates the exact kind of contact and methodology that are effective, while distinguishing between experimentation and behavior modification. He says that behavioral methods are frequently conducted in a manner contrary to the principles of the paradoxical theory of change. There is an implication here that the therapist knows what is good for the client and can provide an anticipated outcome. For example, when I have conducted viva for under-graduate students of psychology in Bangalore, I have often found that many of them use the empty chair within the first five sessions of their internship work with a client. This is concerning as it is often a preplanned, standard operating procedure because they have come to the conclusion that the client needs to do forgiveness work toward the parental figure and only then will they be rid of their anger. However, there is a risk here of emphasizing the client's belief that anger is bad while reinforcing guilt and shame. A dialogic experimental attitude is sensitive to the client's cultural beliefs, values the client's frame of reference, and allows the intersubjective field to creatively direct the therapeutic work.

The experiment is for the client to express trapped feelings, relive past trauma or give voice to the inner child while feeling that they are in a safe space. I think when contact, awareness, experiment, safe emergency and creative adjustment are stressed, then it supports the recovery of past memories as well as hopes and fears for the future, in the here and now. This facilitates a dynamic recreation and chance for assimilation through the use of an experiment (*PHG*,1951).

Adhering to Paradoxical Theory of Change

An important GT concept to keep in mind while conducting an experiment is the paradoxical theory of change. It states that the more we try to change something, the deeper its hold will be on us. Awareness and acceptance of oneself is the only way out of the conundrum of self-criticism and shame because when we accept ourselves for who we are then, there is a possibility for natural change to occur. This is diametrically opposite to the generally held belief that to get cured, people should be wanting to and working toward behavioral change. GT's paradoxical theory of change rests on the premise that 'Change occurs when one becomes what he is, not when he tries to become what he is not' (Beisser, 1970, p. 1). When someone identifies, owns and accepts their being that encompasses their feelings, sensations, thinking and actions, rather than constantly trying to change themselves, it promotes natural growth and opposing this leads to inner conflict and stagnation (Yontef & Schulz, 2016).

Phenomenological Stance

The phenomenological method emphasizes the need for the therapist to be aware of one's own subjectivity, a priori assumptions and biases and to practice 'epoche' (bracketing), in order to be open to new knowledge and experiences. Discussing experimentation with a phenomenological attitude, Yontef and Schulz (2016) say that existential phenomenology does not propose that bias can be eliminated completely and that what can be bracketed is the belief that what one knows is the objective truth. Another way of explaining this is through the concept advocated by the famous romantic poet Samuel T. Coleridge (2010), which he called a willing 'suspension of disbelief' for the moment that sets aside preconceptions and is faithful to the phenomenological experience.

According to Yontef and Schulz (2016),

> Relational GT is a system in which truth is always contextual, perspectival, probabilistic, and corrigible. Relational GT is built on the epistemology of existential phenomenology, which attempts to understand human existence and consciousness. It studies the process of awareness in an attempt to distinguish between actual experience, assumptions, and expectations. The phenomenological method is the foundation for the integration of dialogue and experiment.
>
> *p. 13*

Courage to Stay with the Unknown

A GT experiment is a co-created experience that emerges from the intersubjective field between the therapist and client. Since it is not a manualized or a preconstructed technique, it can be unpredictable. The most productive experiments are what emerges organically in the lived space of the therapy room and seamlessly fit into the dialogic process, and this implies that the therapist does not know nor can guarantee a preordained outcome. This can often be as scary for the therapist as it is for the client, because as human beings we want to be in control of the outcome and uncertainty scares us. Yet as Gestalt therapists, we need to develop the muscle for abiding by the unpredictable and staying with the unknown.

Mindfulness to Culture

Before suggesting an elaborate experiment like twin chair or enactments, the therapist needs to be sure that a good enough therapeutic relationship has been established with the client. Experiments can easily trigger fears of loss of control, anxieties about vulnerability, shame around being seen by the therapist/others in the group setting, and dread of revisiting a painful event. For example, making a client do empty chair for expression of hostile feelings toward a parental figure is likely to backfire especially if the alliance hasn't formed sufficiently. Even if there's a good enough bond, expressing aggression toward an authority figure can be quite stressful for many Indians, especially so when the individual is a woman, lower in the caste hierarchy and a religious minority. Generally, Indians have a deep sense of filial piety and expressing hostile feelings can be accompanied by strong feelings of fear, guilt and shame. It's important to lay the groundwork for a safe situation, sustain contact and establish a fairly secure dialogic relationship with the client before suggesting major experiments that can possibly threaten the client's cultural values.

The above points are some basic considerations for therapists to keep in mind if they want to embed experimentation into a dialogic attitude. I have given below some examples of different experiments and how this approach can be used creatively in a GGT setting. I would recommend these be used judiciously, modified based on the individual client's unique presentations, and with creativity by the therapist to generate experiments as they emerge in the moment. For example, in the last decade or so, I rarely use empty chair in its original form of talking to an empty chair where the client imagines a parent is sitting. When I do use it, I usually ask the client what they imagine might happen if their mother were present and they could express their disappointment to her. I may ask questions like, 'How do you imagine her responding?' and 'What feelings are you experiencing when you imagine her responding like that?' I agree with Mann (2010) that agreement should be reached between the therapist and client, and the experiment should be suitably arranged, meaning that the experiment needs to be enough of a stretch for the client without being too much of a leap. For additional understanding, I recommend that therapists read the *PHG* book and practice some of the experiments given for building self-awareness for the therapist.

Types of Experiments

The experiments compiled below are an integration of what Gestalt practitioners have suggested or have done with their clients in the past (*PHG*, 1951; Brownell, 2010; Yontef & Schulz, 2016; Mann, 2010) and they have been further illuminated with examples from my work. Experiments can be dramatic enactments or exaggerations of emotions; however, the success of the experiment is based on increased awareness for the client and the opening up of creative possibilities of being in the world. Some of the most effective experiments are the simplest, such as encouraging a client to stay with an uncomfortable feeling, developing a small movement made by the client, or encouraging them to try out a different posture (Mann, 2010).

Reflective Experiments

These can be simple relaxation exercises or expressions of stream of consciousness of thoughts, sensations and emotions that flow through one's body and mind. A formal meditation might serve as an experiment, especially if it focuses on spontaneous experience rather than the performance or ability to do meditation. I sometimes use this in the early stages of group formation either as a silent form of reflection or sometimes as an activity, depending on my sense of the group. On occasion, I use the 'rosebush activity' (Allan, 1988; Birch & Carmichael, 2009), and sometimes I use my own personal variations of it depending on how active my muses are. The rosebush is a Jungian play activity designed for children and it works quite well with adults. It invites the members to imagine themselves as a rosebush and make a drawing of it. This is accompanied with inviting them to imagine what kind of a rosebush they are and their location in the environment. I ask the members to share in the larger group if they are comfortable doing so, and if everyone wants to share, then time is dedicated for that. I have found this activity consistently generates awareness for the individual as well as other group members, especially during the processing of individual pieces of art. Each time and with each group, universal as well as unique individual themes emerge. Location of being in a vase inside a house, a garden outside, a fence around the rosebush, no thorns or huge thorns, a creeper on a church wall, fantasies around who nurtures the plant, earthworms, butterflies, sunlight, rain, and presence and absence of other plants nearby often direct toward each member's unique ERTs. Universal themes that emerge are often around isolation, death, meaninglessness, freedom and feelings of helplessness and entrapment. This activity opens up creative possibilities of viewing self and others.

Simple Awareness

According to Yontef and Schulz (2016), certain questions and explorations during the therapeutic dialogue are experiments that help facilitate awareness into the way the client thinks, acts, feels, senses and behaves and how this works for them. The examples given by them are: clarifying and sharpening awareness, bringing into focal awareness what was peripheral before, bringing awareness to what has been kept out of awareness, bringing awareness to what interrupts awareness and experimenting with novel ways of thinking and behaving. I would recommend therapists read this article by Yontef and Schulz (2016) to further their understanding of dialogically and incrementally facilitating awareness.

An example from a therapy group is given below of a young man named Sam who lived in a joint family until adult life and his job led him to relocate to Bangalore city where he lived in a shared accommodation. Sam was a member of a group I worked with across the duration of two years. When he joined the group, he was struggling with a deep sense of inadequacy, difficulty regulating emotions and feelings of isolation. He found it difficult to sustain personal, romantic and work relationships. Over the time span of his being part of the group, I worked with him using small experiments before moving into complex ones, based on his experiences of safety with me and the group. The following is a dialogue between Sam and me during the mid-phase of group therapy:

VA: Tell me more about this inner voice that's critical, can you give voice to that?

SAM: Well, it's this incessant voice in my head that keeps on saying that I am worthless and I keep failing at whatever I take up (is unable to enact the critical voice).

VA: As you are talking about this, your breathing changed, something seems to be holding you back [...] what's happening to you now?

SAM: It's like someone is pushing me, you know it's a barrage of attacks that's choking me [...] I feel constricted in my chest and throat. It's not someone [...] it's my father, uncles and cousins who would attack me and tease me from the time I was small [...] there was no escaping them [...] and there was no way I could say anything to them [...]

VA: I am sorry that happened to you, I imagine you must have felt frightened as a child, scared and powerless to cope with the attacks you experienced [...]

SAM: (tears up and then stops abruptly [...])

VA: Sam? What's happening to you now? [...] you are no longer looking at any of the group members and me [...]

SAM: I was remembering how much I would get punished and bullied if I would tell my mother that they were troubling me, boys aren't supposed to cry and go running to their mothers [...] and it wasn't OK to say I am angry with my father, he did a lot to take care of the family [...] so one day I just stopped complaining [...]

VA: I get this picture of a boy being almost choked by a group of men [...] shamed at seeking protection from your mother, feeling disloyal [...] frightened and alone [...] I wonder what it would be like if I came and sat in the chair beside you?

SAM: (looking at the therapist, starts crying again) [...] yes, I would like that [...] that's how it felt, like they were all sitting on my chest [...] (pauses for a while and then looks at me before continuing) I feel easier to breathe now that you are sitting here [...] not too close but not too far [...] I missed having that with my mother [...]

VA: Well, I am relieved to hear you express the closeness that is comfortable for you [...] You looked at me now after a long while [...] how was that?

SAM: I was feeling bad [...] ashamed earlier sharing this [...] but now it's a little less [...] I don't see rejection and dislike in your eyes [...] you know

I feel disappointed with my mother that she wasn't understanding and didn't protect me [...] I still can't look at others in this group [...]

VA: Yes, I see your disappointment [...] you really wished that at least your mother would keep you safe and be accepting [...] would you want to look at others and maybe hear from them how they feel?

Until this experiment, Sam and the group members had difficulty connecting with each other. However, the understanding the group members developed, toward his vulnerabilities, helped create a space for Sam to reduce his feelings of isolation over time as well as grow closer to them. Other group members narrated their own experiences with abuse and shaming by extended family members, which helped Sam feel that he was not alone in his experience. Some members shared their anger with their mothers who couldn't offer protection in their childhood. To some extent, the strong knots of filial piety weakened a bit both for Sam and other members as he continued his work.

Imagination and Visualization

Mental experiments might be used to explore and visualize a past event that is dread-filled or traumatic or to imagine a future that is hoped for or feared. For example, I remember my therapist taking me through a future visualization when I was feeling great despair about completing my PhD. At that time, I was struggling with raising three kids, of whom one was a toddler; my work; training for certification in Transactional Analysis; and the requirements of the PhD, which were quite rigorous. As I started visualizing all my responsibilities and commitments while juggling them, my therapist asked me to try dropping some and picking up things I really wanted to hold. As the visualization progressed, I felt an excitement while forming the mental images: sensory experiences of what I saw, heard, felt and the way I moved in my future as my PhD culminated in the certification. And when it actually happened two years later, I was startled by how proximal the real experience was to what I had imagined with my therapist.

When I use imaginative experiments with clients or in groups, I invite them to visualize the scenarios that they hope for or dread. In one instance, a group member imagined being a deeply rooted tree in relation to an intimate partner who was nearby but lacking roots. She was stuck between wanting to hold on to the partner but feeling frustrated by his inability to be sturdy and dependable. Further explorations led to her wishing that the tree he represented be removed by her friends. She became startlingly aware of her fear of losing this relationship and wishing for someone else to take control in making a decision about breaking up—a nascent wish for ongoing support until she was able to move herself from her stuck rootedness and a probable struggle with a sense of agency.

Exploration of Polarities

As human beings, we all struggle with the polarities in our lives. These can be universal and existential struggles like: isolation/togetherness, agency/thrownness, death/life and meaning/meaninglessness. In addition, there are individual themes around polarities like strength/vulnerability, love/hate, acceptance/rejection, pride/shame and so on. These polarities can be explored to gain awareness into the rejected or feared parts and how they affect the client interpersonally. The controversial and often misused, yet powerful 'twin chair' can be used to illuminate the polarized parts or voices within the client. For example, in one of the groups a member had reported frequent backache and wanted to dialogue with her body about what it was trying to convey. As they imagined this conversation, what emerged was a voice that said they needed to be strong and responsible always, 'sitting and relaxing is not an option, you need to be strong and keep working hard [...]', and the back saying, 'I am tired, fed up, I don't want to be strong anymore, I want to be weak [...] please get off my back [...]'.

Family Sculpting or Constellation

I use this at times in group therapy if the member requests this, and at times I invite them to try it out, especially if I sense that family sculpting would support the member to understand the family dynamics experienced as a child, and that are now interrupting living their life fully. Based on the individual member's comfort, volunteers are selected to play the roles of significant figures and the client sculpts and directs the members toward the role. When there is sufficient attunement in the group, this experiment can be very powerful in the way it unfolds, create a field in the present here and now of client's childhood experiences, and facilitate awareness in the client about his present internal and interpersonal conflicts. In addition, it helps the group members develop deep intimate connections to each other in the group.

Finally, given below is a story narrated by a group member who has been given the name Alekya, an Indian name meaning 'something that cannot be written' or 'a great warrior'. She was a trainee in one of the training groups I conducted over three years as well as the residential group therapy that I conduct annually (for the last six years). I am grateful to Alekya for sharing her experiences, which includes some of the experiments I used with her within a group setting. The 'coin' experiment she has described below is an imaginative technique that evolved during the work with Alekya to build awareness into the weight of shame that both of us felt was familial as well as cultural.

My Journey with Shame: Alekya's Story

Group therapy using a Gestalt approach has had a big impact on my personal growth. I wished to share my journey through the group process that I have been a part of, so I went back to looking at my experiences and where I was around six years back. I noticed shame sitting right in the center of my field. A lot of shame ... shame that blocked me, shame that made me feel small, shame that kept me out of awareness of who I am. Did I recognize it early on? No!

I remember my first encounter with it was during one of the practice sessions in the training group where my facilitator said I stopped the client too early. Shame hit me, telling me, how could I miss this? What would the group members think of me? Such a bad counselor I am! I promised subtly to myself that it's best not to volunteer to be a counselor during practice sessions—readily gulping down the judgment I had created for myself. Cautiously I entered into another training and experiential group where I took the role of the client more often. Alas! My strategy didn't work at all. As I was working with my issues, I kept calling my ex-partner 'my husband', and during the feedback one of my peers pointed out, 'I noticed while you were saying that he is still wanting the relationship, you kept saying "my husband", what does it mean?' I was taken aback. Shame came right on my face—my paradox, where the more I wanted to be away from the past relationship, the more I got stuck with it. This was visible to everybody and I wondered if something was not OK with me that I carry this level of shame.

Soon I realized there is no hiding from shame in a group space. I could see my peers also struggling with this emotion as they narrated their experiences. Shame of failing in life, of breaking down, of making mistakes, of not being who they wanted to be, of not being better, of being absent for the self ... everything I carried within myself would come up, if not for me, then for my peers. And it would become hard to not connect with it when the group facilitator would ask me, 'what's happening to you?' The support to face shame started changing something existentially in me. The safety my group offered to me and the holding I received from the group facilitator helped me engage with the wall I had created to hide my shame. For me, having a nonjudgmental space, an audience that was interested in revisiting my pain with me, a space that reassured me that I will be accepted, loved and valued, irrespective of what I do in life, was fundamental to moving past the wall.

My first breakthrough happened when I decided to open up the shame I carry as a mother toward a daughter who was born with a congenital heart defect. For years I had felt guilty that there was a time when I considered aborting the baby due to medical reasons. At one point, I blamed her birth for bringing a huge debt for the family. Lately, I felt responsible for not being there for her emotionally post her medical recovery. To my surprise, after hearing me, rather than questioning me, or judging me for being this kind of mother, the group and the facilitator shared the grief, frustration, loneliness and the exhaustion they experienced while I narrated my story. It was unbelievable for me that a whole group of people were experiencing my frustration and sadness that I had buried in myself, and could connect with the lack of nurturance I experienced at that stage in my life, the comfort and support I yearned for during this tough phase *of my life. I always denied grieving for my loss because like all the others in my family and friends, saving my daughter was the mission. Who really cared for the mother who got lost in that mission? Nobody had ever cried for that mother … I had never cried for me … **Crying with this group for me was the beginning of my grieving**.*

*Soon after, an incident of a client withdrawing from therapy suddenly generated a lot of shame in me. The thought of what my peers will think, will they give me a chance to explain, or have I harmed the client … these were the thoughts that came to my mind. Nothing soothed me enough until I brought it to the group space. Assurances of trust in my work from the group didn't let me come back to normalcy. It was too much to handle and it was too much in my body! My facilitator invited me to an experimentation … she collected a lot of coins together from group members and asked me to divide the coins in parts to symbolically represent how much shame goes to each share. I had many—society, gender, self, family, workspace—something kept changing in me when I was dividing the coins. My breath changed, my abdomen freed up a bit, I was feeling less shaken. She helped me eliminate familial and cultural shame by asking what's mine and not mine, what I would want to keep and what I would discard, and segregating which parts of my life were receiving a larger share of shame from other sources, such as my mother from her own female lineage. It was a moving experience to say, 'this is not my share, it's others" and moving closer to what's mine. It was an experience of an unwanted load I was carrying—a **load of mine and others'**. I felt lighter by segregating the coins.*

Finally resting on my load alone, which was closely connected to what I have received from my mother and internalized strongly. Everything was shamed in my world. If I asked something, it was shameful because I am so dumb; if my marriage didn't work, it was shameful because it's me who didn't know how to hold it like others do; if I felt overwhelmed with kids, it's because I indulged them more than needed. I learned to stay submerged in the weight of shame rather than throwing it away and saying it's not mine.

The group sharing with me how they too felt the burden of my shame, and how they felt moved with my pain of facing this burden alone, touched me. My facilitator asking me to keep the share of coins that I was not ready to give up was an honoring experience as it told me it was OK to not immediately deal with everything that comes up, rather than feeling shamed for not being ready.

I wondered if these incidental exchanges were good enough to heal me, someone who has carried a lot of trauma since childhood? Was the load of shame small enough to be reduced with these coins, or would I need to face it more directly?

An opportunity to directly work with shame came up in one of the residential retreats. We had to write our story of any incident as a third person and share it in the group, and I chose to narrate the experience of child sexual abuse that I underwent at the age of 11. The memory of this incident is deep seated and I have carried a huge shame inside me regarding it. I struggled to make a choice as to how the group can help me with this ... with what's so much a part of my existence ... part of my family system.

*Invitation to participate in a family sculpting by the group facilitator took me toward exploring it. My frozen family system that failed to respond at every level for each one of us—my parents abandoning us, my father abandoning my mother, my siblings abandoning me—**the chain looked too strong to break**. During the process, I felt like I was reaching for the same door that I had been knocking on all these years and returning empty-handed and hurt. Something was very powerful about this visual of seeing my group members enact the role of my family frozen there and the door being locked very strongly. In hindsight, the idea of writing a traumatic incident as the story of another person and narrating it in the group was the start of an empowering experience. It healed me as I shared something hidden so deep in me—so old, so complicated—with an empathetic audience ready to own roles from my life, bring themselves into my pain, access their own emotions to hold mine, and willingness to be impacted by what came up ... a courage maybe my family never had, and a witness I always yearned for to heal my pain ... a witness who saw me.*

My journey with Gestalt group therapy is an ongoing one. Over the years, the engagement with shame has opened up a lot within me. I call it the Gestalt that stayed in my field so much that unless I saw it enough, it refused to give permission to let any other Gestalt take center stage in my life. Now I have some awareness of where I have been stuck. Shame visits me infrequently nowadays and she sits comfortably in my prayer corner. Whenever I see her, I welcome her because every time she visits, I know she is triggering some need in me to see something that I haven't. I have recently realized that often my shame accompanies helplessness, a feeling that has troubled me very much. A state of helplessness that triggers shame, and which dictates my internal state and decisions.

I welcome the new Gestalt arriving in my field.

References

Allan, J. A. B. (1988). *Inscapes of the child's world: Jungian counseling in schools and clinics*. Spring Publications.

Beisser, A. (1970). The paradoxical theory of change. *Gestalt Therapy Now*. www.gest alt.org/arnie.htm

Birch, J., & Carmichael, K. D. (2009). Using drawings in play therapy: A Jungian approach. *Alabama Counseling Association Journal, 34*(2), 2–7.

Brownell, P. (2010). *Gestalt therapy: A guide to contemporary practice*. Springer.

Coleridge, S. T. (2010). Samuel Taylor Coleridge (1772–1834). In V. B. Leitch, W. E. Cain, L. A. Finke, & B. E. Johnson (Eds.), *The Norton anthology of theory and criticism* (pp. 677–682). W. W. Norton.

Fogarty, M., Bhar, S., Theiler, S., & O'Shea, L. (2016). What do gestalt therapists do in the clinic? The expert consensus. *British Gestalt Journal, 25*(1), 32–41.

Greenberg, L. S., & Kahn, S. E. (1978). Experimentation: A gestalt approach to counselling. *Canadian Journal of Counselling and Psychotherapy, 13*(1), 23–27.

Hycner, R. H. (1985). Dialogical gestalt therapy: An initial proposal. *Gestalt Journal, 8*(1), 23–49.

Jacobs, L. (1989). Dialogue in gestalt theory and therapy. *Gestalt Journal, 12*(1), 25–67.

Mann, D. (2010). *Gestalt therapy: 100 key points and techniques*. Routledge.

Melnick, J. (1980). The use of therapist-imposed structure in gestalt therapy. *Gestalt Journal, 3*(2), 4–20.

Melnick, J., & Nevis, S. M. (1997). Diagnosing in the here and now: The experience cycle and DSM IV. *British Gestalt Journal, 6*(2), 97–106.

Perls, F. S., Hefferline, R. E., & Goodman, P. (1951). *Gestalt therapy: Excitement and growth in the human personality*. Dell.

Perls, L. (1992). Concepts and misconceptions of gestalt therapy. *Journal of Humanistic Psychology, 32*(3), 50–56. https://doi.org/10.1177/0022167892323004

Polster, M. (2005). Gestalt terapie: Vyvoj a vyuziti. In J. K. Zeig (Ed.), *Uměni psychoterapie* (pp. 516–532). Portál.

Roubal, J. (2009). Experiment: A creative phenomenon of the field. *Gestalt Review, 13*(3), 263–276. https://doi.org/10.5325/gestaltreview.13.3.0263

Roubal, J. (2019). An experimental approach: Follow by leading. In P. Brownell (Ed.), *Handbook for theory, research, and practice in gestalt therapy* (pp. 220–267). Cambridge Scholars.

Yontef, G. M. (1993). *Awareness, dialogue & process: Essays on gestalt therapy*. Gestalt Journal Press.

Yontef, G. M. (2007). The power of the immediate moment in gestalt therapy. *Journal of Contemporary Psychotherapy, 37*(1), 17–23. https://doi.org/10.1007/s10879-006-9030-0

Yontef, G. M., & Fuhr, R. (2005). Gestalt therapy theory of change. In A. L. Woldt & S. M. Toman (Eds.), *Gestalt therapy: History, theory, and practice.* (pp. 81–100). SAGE.

Yontef, G. M., & Jacobs, L. (2005). Gestalt therapy. In R. J. Corsini & D. Wedding (Eds.), *Current psychotherapies* (pp. 299–336). Thomson Brooks/Cole.

Yontef, G. M., & Schulz, F. (2016). Dialogue and experiment. *British Gestalt Journal, 25*(1), 9–21.

Conclusion

This book was influenced by my earliest memories of living in my village, being a curious witness to my grandfather's tea groups, grandmother's village bathing pond groups, and watching the temple theater plays with my mother, grandmother and our village community. Witnessing the communal spirit and the temple festivals has perhaps influenced my beliefs around relationships and the powerful impact of expressing ourselves through our senses and body. The process of growing up, my Western education, the Indian ethos, my Hindu middle-class upbringing, my experiences of groups as a trainee therapist, Pacific Gestalt Institute exposure, and my experiences of leading groups have combined to draw this book closer to wholeness. The essence of who I am has evolved, and continues to, in my relational field.

I hope as you continued to read this book, the importance of relationality, groups and communities became more meaningful for you. In a professional capacity, I hope this book will add value to the Gestalt community in the world who work with the Indian diaspora or clients who have been profoundly impacted by collectivistic and hierarchical cultural characteristics and colonialism. I hope this book will be influential for mental health practitioners and students of psychology in India for the practical experiences on relationality it has provided.

Moreover, I hope this book will help my colleagues and students in India expand their knowledge about GT that goes beyond techniques like empty chair and toward an in-depth understanding of the rich theoretical underpinning that supports a wholesome practice of GT.

If working with groups excites you, if human potential to heal and change in startling ways inspires you, if bringing the self of the therapist into the relational field motivates you, if you are open to staying with uncertainties, then this book was intended for you. If you are yearning to make meaning of existence and how it isolates us from others while binding us in togetherness, then this book was intended for you. If you have learned more about working sensitively within the Indian cultural context while rethinking our colonial

DOI: 10.4324/9781003348337-11

education, then I hope this book has fulfilled your quest to an approximation. When you decided to pick up this book and started reading it, you entered our group circle of belongingness and I wish you feel welcome. As you put down this book, I hope you are thoughtful about how deeply interwoven your mind, body, emotions and actions are with your environment.

Index

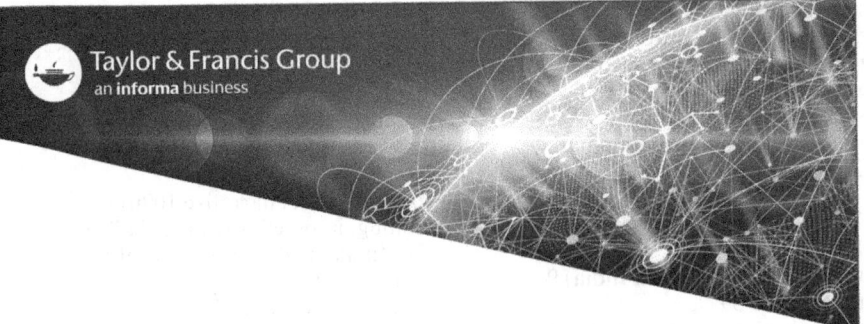
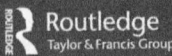
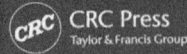